Safeguarding adults and children with disabilities against abuse

Report drawn up by
Professor Hilary Brown

in co-operation with
the Working Group on Violence Against,
and Ill-treatment as well as Abuse
of People with Disabilities

Integration of people with disabilities

Council of Europe Publishing

French edition:

La protection des adultes et enfants handicapés contre les abus

ISBN 92-871-4918-6

Cover design: Graphic Design Workshop, Council of Europe
Layout: Desktop Publishing Unit, Council of Europe

Edited by Council of Europe Publishing
http://book.coe.int
F-67075 Strasbourg Cedex

ISBN 92-871-4919-4
© Council of Europe, February 2003
Printed at the Council of Europe

4 BRo

CONTENTS

EXECUTIVE SUMMARY

About the report

This report addresses a broad range of abuses and mistreatment committed against all disabled children and adults. It has been prepared by Professor Hilary Brown, Consultant, in co-operation with the Council of Europe Working Group on Violence Against, and Ill-treatment as well as Abuse of People with Disabilities (Partial Agreement in the Social and Public Health field). In defining abuse the group was mindful that discrimination against people with disabilities is inextricably linked to abuse and that they are often offered less support than other people and barred from effective means of escape or redress when they are harmed. The report aims to make visible the extent and nature of such abuse and to ensure that people with disabilities are safeguarded against deliberate and/or avoidable harm at least to the same extent as other citizens and that where they are especially vulnerable additional measures are put in place to assure their safety.

This document sets out :

- a workable definition of violence, abuse, mistreatment and neglect;
- case studies to show how these issues affect the lives of people with disabilities;
- an overview of research and sources of information on these issues;
- information to help professionals assess risk to people with disabilities;
- a brief account of how these issues are being addressed by member countries;

- examples of good practice in policy and service development; and

- an outline of the role of public and non-governmental organisations in response to issues of abuse in the lives of people with disabilities.

Defining abuse

The report provides a working definition of abuse that includes physical and sexual abuse, psychological harm, financial abuse and neglect/abandonment whether physical or emotional. It addresses abuse in all settings with a particular concern for people still living in closed institutions and for those abused by people in positions of authority. It is concerned with the failure to give disabled people access to equivalent health care. Special concern is voiced for those who are doubly disadvantaged including women and girls with disabilities and disabled people from ethnic and refugee communities or from war-torn countries. The report considers capacity and consent as key issues in determining whether acts are abusive or whether they represent valid choices made by disabled people whose rights to make decisions and take risks are equal to those of other citizens. The scope of concerns include:

- seriously inadequate care and attention to basic needs including nutrition, health care and access to educational and social opportunities;

- individual acts of cruelty or sexual aggression by persons who are in the role of care givers;

- breaches of civil liberties such as incarceration without due process, "enforced cohabitation" in group homes or institutions, prohibition of sexual relationships or marriage, lack of privacy or intrusion into or interruption of mail or telephone calls or visits in institutional or family settings and/or continued isolation from sources of support or advocacy;

- acts of bullying or random violence within community settings, some of which may represent more extreme forms of generally held prejudice against people with disabilities or, of greater concern, global ideologies which are inimical to disabled persons;

- practice by individual staff which falls well outside, or below, accepted professional norms;
- abuses by other service users within service settings where attention has not been paid to safe groupings or sufficient supervision to ensure safe placements;
- authorised treatments and interventions which are not in the person's best interests and/or which rest on an inaccurate or incomplete understanding of their condition and needs, for example punitive responses to challenging behaviour, seclusion, unconsented ECT, or aversive behavioural programmes.

Abuse is defined as:

Any act, or failure to act, which results in a significant breach of a vulnerable person's human rights, civil liberties, bodily integrity, dignity or general well-being, whether intended or inadvertent, including sexual relationships or financial transactions to which the person has not or cannot validly consent, or which are deliberately exploitative. Abuse may be perpetrated by any person (including by other people with disabilities) but it is of special concern when it takes place within a relationship of trust characterised by powerful positions based on:

- legal, professional or authority status;

- unequal physical, economic or social power;

- responsibility for the person's day-to-day care;

- and/or inequalities of gender, race, religion or sexual orientation.

It may arise out of individual cruelty, inadequate service provision or society's indifference.

It requires a proportional response – one which does not cut across valid choices made by individuals with disabilities but one which does recognise vulnerability and exploitation.

An overview of research

The report offers an overview of research and urges governments to collaborate in generating comparable data. Disabled
children and adults should be identified within statistics generated routinely about crime and child/adult protection interventions. While it is impossible to establish exact figures for
incidence (number of reports in a given time span) or **prevalence** (percentage of disabled people abused at some time
during their lifetime) or for raised levels of risk, it is possible
to say that disabled people are exposed to at least the same
and probably more risk of abuse as other people and that they
require at least the same level of protection and access to
redress.

A consensus exists in the literature that the risks of abuse are
exacerbated by:

• public hostility or indifference to people who are visibly different;

• institutional cultures, regimes and structures in which direct
care staff have low skills, status and pay; where there is
resistance to change and a closed community; unequal pay,
conditions and training opportunities for qualified and
unqualified staff;

• repeated exposure to multiple carers for those in receipt of
personal assistance and intimate care;

• ignorance and poor training of staff who work with people
who have complex needs and/or challenging behaviours;

• lack of regulation or strong accountability to an independent agency/department.

Data from inquiries and service evaluation also throw light on
the dynamics which lead to abuse and the possibilities for
remediation. User involvement in planning and conducting
research is urged as is international collaboration in funding
and design of research programmes and scholarly exchange.

The legal framework

The legal framework and enforcement process plays an important part in the protection of disabled people by enshrining rights and safeguards in legislation and by providing important avenues through which disabled people can seek redress. Specific offences set clear boundaries around what is acceptable and may provide additional safeguards for the most vulnerable people. The law also provides the basis for the involvement of the state by defining (and limiting) the powers and the duties of public bodies to intervene in the lives of individual citizens.

The European Convention on Human Rights sets out these principles:

- formal *equality* of disabled children and adults and entitlement to *equivalent* treatment in law and health care with whatever assistance they need to pursue and uphold this;

- *proportionality* and independent *scrutiny* of any controlling, protective or limiting approaches, for example where detention or restraint is thought to be in the best interests of a disabled person and/or necessary to secure their immediate safety or the protection of others, or where disabled people might be considered to be at risk of exploitation and unable to consent to certain transactions.

These protections work at different levels, in relation to:

- the *definition* of abuse against disabled people through the use of generic criminal codes and where laws specify cir cumstances or acts which are illegal in relation to disabled people, for example sexual or financial exploitation;

- the part that law plays in *prevention* of abuse either directly or by setting up safeguards in services which make abuse of disabled people less likely. This law includes for example, legislation about the standards and regulation of professionals and care settings; and/or legal processes to evaluate the use of unwarranted force or detention and a framework to limit or mandate the appropriate sharing of information;

- access to the criminal or civil law to provide *redress* and/or compensation to disabled people who have been victims of violence and to punish wrongdoers which, in itself, sends important signals that the community values disabled people and will act to protect them. Access to justice is an important element of civil liberties and redress should be available through ordinary routes with additional assistance where this is necessary such as in helping individuals to give evidence in court and to participate in the legal process without being intimidated (see Home Office 1998; European Disability Forum (EDF) 1999a:14-5).

The legal systems of member states vary considerably, some drawing on an inquisitorial, and others an adversarial tradition but the report offers a series of pointers and models to assist member states in reviewing their own legislation in order to identify gaps and priorities. It also notes that judges, police officers, probation officers and other professionals working within the criminal justice system have considerable training needs if they are to begin to offer a more inclusive and less discriminatory approach to disabled people whether as victims, witnesses or offenders or as applicants under civil law to have their rights upheld.

Examples of prevention in action

The report provides examples of work that is being done to strengthen protection for individuals both within specific social care agencies and in a broader social context. Intervention is needed at different *stages:* at the *primary* stage which prevents abuse from happening at all, at a *secondary* stage to ensure that abuse is promptly identified and referred to appropriate agencies who will intervene to stop it recurring and at the *tertiary* stage to treat individuals who have been abused and help them to recover without sustaining long-term problems related to trauma and distress. Action is also needed at different *levels,* with individuals directly but also through structural change. A third dimension is the *orientation* of the intervention: in relation to abuse a *defensive (reactive)* strategy would be one which seeks to avert danger, for example through screening out unsuitable staff, whereas an *offensive (proactive)* strategy will tackle risks by promoting positives through for example enhancing user involvement, improving key areas of practice or implementing quality assurance programmes.

The report collates a number of initiatives from member states including programmes ranging from sexual education and assertiveness training to policy documents setting out how agencies should work together to investigate concerns, arrangements for receiving complaints and for inspecting services and the development of resources to provide therapeutic support to people who have been abused.

Conclusion

The report makes visible a broad range of harm and mistreatment, which occurs across a range of settings and circumstances. It advocates a model of protection that enhances the rights of disabled children and adults to take decisions and appropriate risks in their ordinary lives. The groups's recommendations provide an achievable agenda for action at all levels against which progress can be measured. Work to protect children and adults with disabilities in our communities is an important commitment that sits alongside, and may be seen as part of, the Council of Europe's broader agenda on integration and social inclusion of people with disabilities.

PREFACE

The Council of Europe

The Council of Europe is a political organisation which was founded on 5 May 1949 by ten European countries in order to promote greater unity between its members. It now numbers 44 member states[1].

The main aims of the Organisation are to reinforce democracy, human rights and the rule of law and to develop common responses to political, social, cultural and legal challenges in its member states. Since 1989 the Council of Europe has integrated most of the countries of central and eastern Europe into its structures and supported them in their efforts to implement and consolidate their political, legal and administrative reforms.

The European Court of Human Rights is the judicial body competent to adjudicate complaints brought against a state by individuals, associations or other contracting states on grounds of violation of the European Convention on Human Rights.

Partial Agreement in the Social and Public Health Field

Where a lesser number of member states of the Council of Europe wish to engage in some action in which not all their

---

1. Albania, Andorra, Armenia, Austria, Azerbaijan, Belgium, Bosnia and Herzogovina, Bulgaria, Croatia, Cyprus, Czech Republic, Denmark, Estonia, Finland, France, Georgia, Germany, Greece, Hungary, Iceland, Ireland, Italy, Latvia, Liechtenstein, Lithuania, Luxembourg, Malta, Moldova, The Netherlands, Norway, Poland, Portugal, Romania, Russian Federation, San Marino, Slovak Republic, Slovenia, Spain, Sweden, Switzerland, "the former Yugoslav Republic of Macedonia", Turkey, Ukraine, United Kingdom of Great Britain and Northern Ireland.

European partners desire to join, they can conclude a 'Partial Agreement' which is binding on themselves alone.

The Partial Agreement in the Social and Public Health Field was concluded on this basis in 1959. At present, the Partial Agreement in the Social and Public Health Field has 18 member states.[1]

The principal areas of activity are:

- rehabilitation and integration of people with disabilities;
- protection of public health and especially the health of the consumer.

The activities in the sphere of rehabilitation are supervised by the Committee on the Rehabilitation and Integration of People with disabilities and guided by the Coherent policy for people with disabilities, adopted by the Committee of Ministers of the Council of Europe in 1992 as Recommendation No. R (92) 6. The Partial Agreement is committed to upholding the rights of people with disabilities and advocates for their integration and full participation in society. Such a commitment should also be seen against the background of the European Convention on Human Rights and the European Social Charter, both major instruments of the Council of Europe.

The present report and recommendations have been pre-pared by Professor Hilary Brown, consultant, in co-operation with the Working group on violence against and ill-treatment as well as abuse of people with disabilities, a sub-group of the Committee on the Rehabilitation and Integration of People with disabilities. Special thanks are due to the United Kingdom Department of Health and the Salomons Centre for Applied Social and Psychological Development, Canterbury University College, for having made Professor Brown available for this project.

---

1. Austria, Belgium, Cyprus, Denmark, Finland, France, Germany, Ireland, Italy, Luxembourg, The Netherlands, Norway, Portugal, Slovenia, Spain, Sweden, Switzerland, United Kingdom of Great Britain and Northern Ireland.

1. INTRODUCTION

1.1. The Council of Europe against abuse

The Council of Europe has addressed abuse in several arenas of its work. Recommendations and reports have already been issued regarding child and elder abuse, violence in the family, sexual abuse, violence against women, violence in schools, racist and xenophobic violence as well as ill-treatment in closed institutions. Training workshops and awareness raising campaigns have also been conducted on many of these topics. Furthermore, the European Committee for the Prevention of Torture and Inhuman or Degrading Treatment or Punishment (CPT) makes regular visits to prisons, detention centres and psychiatric institutions in order to examine the treatment of persons deprived of their liberty.

Due to mounting concerns about violence perpetrated against people with disabilities in particular, a working group on violence against and ill-treatment as well as abuse of people with disabilities was set up in 1998 by the Committee on the Rehabilitation and Integration of People with disabilities (Partial Agreement in the Social and Public Health Field). The working group met in Strasbourg on five occasions between 1999-2001. The members of the group are listed in the appendix. The terms of reference of the group were the following:

a. to define and evaluate the problem of violence against, and ill-treatment as well as abuse of children and adults within and outside institutions, covering people with the whole range of disabilities, but excluding the issue of discrimination;

b. to analyse information about relevant legislation and its implementation, policies and strategies at international and national level, taking into account the work of other groups, within and outside the Council of Europe, and the perspective of people with disabilities, their families and carers, and including consideration of the following:

i. preventing and combating violence, ill-treatment and abuse in all situations by raising public awareness, promoting open discussion, and improving professional education, training, in-service support and guidance;

ii. improving detection and reporting of violence, ill-treatment and abuse in all situations;

iii. focusing on practical measures, guidelines and strategies rather than on a comparative analysis of statistical data;

c. to submit a first series of concrete recommendations to the Committee on the Rehabilitation and Integration of People with disabilities (CD-P-RR).

The present report aims to complete the terms of reference of the group. It has been drafted by Professor Hilary Brown, Consultant to the working group, in the context of the group's meetings. The group collected data and collated information of recent research in member states and from North America and then worked through debate and discussion of a series of drafts of this report. Organisations representing people with disabilities, their families and carers were consulted through hearings, written consultations and in the context of the European Union Day of Disabled Persons of 1999, which focused on the theme of violence and abuse against people with disabilities. Delegates consulted widely within their own countries to collect case studies and identify examples of good practice.

A number of related documents have been referred to in the course of drafting this report. A list is included in the References section at the end of the document.

1.2. A note on terminology

The group spent considerable time discussing the title of this report and the terminology to be used throughout the document. The remit of the working group responsible for this work was originally framed as "violence against, and ill-treatment, as well as abuse of, people with disabilities".

Words are very powerful, especially those which describe wrong-doing, and they become charged with nuances which may be lost in translation. In this report we have interpreted "violence, mistreatment and abuse" broadly taking the following considerations into account:

- Some of these terms are more or less comprehensive and more or less neutral than others: for example force can in certain circumstances be legitimate whereas violence is a more morally loaded term.

- Neglect whether caused by a failure to act, abandonment, or extremes of isolation should be considered alongside acts which cause actual physical harm.

- The intentions of the person responsible for harm alters the interpretation put on behaviour: sexual acts or financial transactions which take place in the context of authority, coercion, deception or exploitation for example give rise to particular concern.

- Informed and valid consent is a key concept in determining whether an act or transaction is abusive and/or whether a disabled person's refusal to accept help should be taken at face value.

- Violations of civil liberties or human rights may take place as a result of structural problems rather than individual cruelty, for example as a result of coercive treatments which might be common-place or legitimated; as a result of institutional regimes; or because state benefits and legal procedures are inflexible or inadequate.

- Abuse takes place against a backdrop of more pervasive unequal treatment: discrimination and social exclusion are viewed as important contributory factors to individual instances of abuse, exploitation and deprivation although they are not the primary focus of this report.

In the United Kingdom the term *abuse* is used to cover this broad range of harmful actions and failures to act in a range of circumstances: it can refer to both abuse *by* an individual as well as abuse *of* a person's human rights and its use in this report is designed to simplify the text where multiple meanings are intended. Its use is not designed to disguise or minimise the severity of violent or criminal acts perpetrated against people with disabilities.

What is important is that people with disabilities are safeguarded against deliberate and/or avoidable harm at least to the same extent as other citizens and that where they are especially vulnerable additional measures are put in place to assure their safety.

1.3. Who is included within the term "people with disabilities"?

This report refers to all people with disabilities, whether adults or children, including

- people with physical and sensory impairments;
- people with intellectual disabilities and autism;
- mentally ill people;
- people who have drug or alcohol problems;
- people with hidden disabilities and medical conditions such as epilepsy, rheumatism, diabetes and other chronic conditions;
- people with chronic illnesses, which may or may not be terminal, including dementia and Aids related illnesses.

It should be noted that specific policies in member states do not necessarily identify all these people as disabled persons.

The term "people with disabilities" or "disabled people" is somewhat unusually used throughout the report to denote all of these groups but it is used with caution and specific needs and issues are highlighted. This report is primarily concerned with people under the age of 65 but clearly links should be made with older people's services and with elder abuse prevention programmes in member states to ensure that resources and skills are shared appropriately (McCreadie

1996; Study Group on Violence Against Elderly People 1993; AEP 2000). The report is not primarily concerned with the treatment of people with disabilities who commit violent acts themselves, for example as part of a mental illness; but the need to assess risks and safeguard other people using services is acknowledged throughout (AEP 2000).

The term "people with disabilities" is in itself contentious and may be interpreted differently in different member states. Articles 17 and 18 of the United Nations Standard Rules on the Equalization of Opportunities for Persons with Disabilities define disability as the interaction between a person's impairment and their environment. The United Nations document refers to a range of impairments including *"physical, intellectual or sensory impairment, medical conditions or mental illness. Such impairments, conditions or illnesses may be permanent or transitory in nature"*. Many of these groups have taken a "people first" approach to the issue of labelling which importantly recognises that their identity as fellow citizens should take priority over any special needs they may have. People with physical disabilities, drawing on their analysis of a social model of disability (as opposed to a medicalised model) and on a shared identity as disabled persons, often prefer to put their disabled status up-front. It will be seen that since there is no universal consensus across Europe about this question the terms "disabled people" and "people with disabilities" are used interchangeably.

It is important to distinguish between the impact of physical or sensory impairments and intellectual disabilities or mental illness and also to acknowledge varying degrees of severity of different impairments. While adults with physical impairments will usually be able to make decisions for themselves they are often not given adequate practical and financial assistance and access to appropriate information. In contrast, people with significant degrees of intellectual disability may need others to make complex decisions on their behalf as well as to act for them to put these into practice. Mentally ill people, or those with disordered thought states, may move in and out of states of vulnerability and need varying levels of help with decision-making. An undifferentiated approach to disability may mean that individuals are offered inappropriate help and/or that they are burdened with inaccurate stereotypes and accumulated prejudices. Examples include deaf people who complain that they are labelled as "crazy" when they use sign language or people who are depressed who are assumed to have intellectual disabilities because they are temporarily unable to do the things they used to do. People with profound impairments, including those who are unable to communicate, may require very specific safeguards (AEP 2000:2).

1.4. Underlying values relating to empowerment, discrimination and abuse

The "Working group on violence against, and ill-treatment, as well as abuse of, people with disabilities" is a sub-group of the "Committee on the Rehabilitation and Integration of people with disabilities". This locates their work in the context of a range of policies designed to combat discrimination against people with disabilities, to ensure their inclusion in the social and economic life of their communities and to uphold their civil rights. The "Katholieke Vereniging voor Gehandicapten" state these rights as an essential reference point when considering issues of abuse and neglect, namely that:

> "All people with disabilities are entitled to dignity and equal opportunity. This means that they are entitled to their own income, education, employment, acceptance and integration in social life including genuine accessibility, as well as medical and functional rehabilitation". (Note by the Belgian delegation)

This is often referred to as "empowerment" in that it provides people with disabilities with the means to run their own lives and make their own decisions. At face value it might seem as if measures to protect people with disabilities might run counter to this agenda and cut across campaigns to assure autonomy, choice and freedom to take ordinary risks. But there is no suggestion of a protective "blanket" being placed over all people with disabilities. It would be simplistic to suppose that all these groups and individuals are particularly "vulnerable" to abuse or in need of *special* protection or intervention.

For most adults with physical or sensory impairments the task of relevant agencies will be to assure equality of protection through

- creating and supporting positive attitudes and ideologies towards people with disabilities;

- ensuring that service settings are safe and appropriately staffed and that practice is based on respect for the integrity of the person at all times;

- providing formal safeguards in contentious areas of practice such as the use of control, restraint or detention;

- assuring equitable access to the legal system and to public facilities;

- helping people to access support if they have been victimised.

For most people with disabilities the aim is not so much to provide *extra* protection but to ensure that they **are protected at least to the same extent as other citizens,** any of whom may face abuse or exploitation in childhood or as adults. But for some disabled children and adults, especially those with significant intellectual disabilities, a more proactive stance will be needed. Some people with disabilities, at some times in their lives and in some situations, may not be able to make appropriate decisions for themselves or take steps to protect themselves from exploitation, nor will they be able to seek help when they are out of their depth. They may be put at significant risk by "laissez-faire" approaches that downplay the impact of their impairment(s), underestimate the impact of controlling relationships and authority figures or minimise their need for support in managing their affairs. Groups which may be particularly at risk are those with challenging behaviours, severe intellectual disabilities, autism, and/or enduring mental health problems.

There are some advantages and some disadvantages in addressing the issues of disabled children alongside those of disabled adults. Structures for protection of all children are more developed than those for vulnerable adults in most member states. Definitions are more "clear-cut", and the moral imperative to intervene is more clearly established. But disabled children are often marginalized and poorly served within this generic framework. Westcott and Jones (1999) note how earlier studies tended to label children as "abuse provoking" as if the cause lay with them and their impairments rather than within the systems which have grown up to serve them. The task of campaigners is to counter such assumptions and make disabled children visible as a minority group with distinct needs within mainstream child protection processes.

Disabled adults on the other hand, may not be recognized as potential victims of abuse: procedures may not exist to help them make complaints or seek redress, especially if they are harmed within the services that are supposed to be helping them. There may be ambiguity (in law as well as in society at large) about whether intervention is in their best interests, or in what circumstances a disabled person might be making a valid choice to remain in an abusive relationship or setting[1].

Given that many people with disabilities live relatively autonomously within their communities, member states may want to focus protective policies on those most in need of assistance. The English Law Commission has recently suggested a category of "vulnerable adult" being a person over 18 years of age who:

> *"is or may be in need of community care services by reason of mental or other disability, age or illness and who is or may be unable to take care of him or herself or unable to protect him or herself against significant harm or exploitation"* (Law Commission 1995: cmnd 231).

---

1. In this report the term "people with disabilities" or "disabled persons" is used inclusively to embrace both children and adults. Where issues are specific the terms "disabled adults" and "disabled children" are used.

This definition is designed to ensure that issues which arise for physically disabled people will be dealt with in a civil liberties framework and only those more severely impaired persons whose capacity to "protect themselves from serious exploitation or significant harm" is in question, will be offered the help that they need, when they have been, or are at risk of being, abused.[1] This help may include paying attention to the way their services are provided and offering assistance when accessing those safeguards provided through the civil and criminal justice systems of their own countries. Finding a balance between empowerment and protection that works for each individual is a core task for social care agencies.

Any specific legislation or policy guidance introduced in member countries needs to reflect this balance since legislation may otherwise be:

"interpreted as paternalistic and stigmatizing and as encouraging the stereotype that people with disabilities are intrinsically incompetent. It can also deny people with disabilities the natural right to expose themselves to legitimate risks." (European Disability Forum (EDF) 1999a:15)

On the other hand disabled children and adults may be exposed to particular risks because they use services and are in receipt of residential or personal care and hence are placed in unique situations (Westcott & Jones 1999). They may also be subjected to personal violence in their relationships, homes and communities because these are relatively "ordinary" life experiences. The social model of disability holds that an adult or child is only "handicapped" to the extent that "shortcomings in the environment" lead to loss or limitation of opportunities to take part in the life of the community on an equal level with others"[2]. We would argue that a person may also only be vulnerable to the extent that their rights are not

---

1. France also groups various vulnerable groups together placing people with disabilities alongside pregnant women and elderly people as "vulnerable adults." They are then treated at law within the same framework as abused children.
2. Article 17 and 18 of the United Nation Standard Rules on the Equalisation of Opportunities for Persons with Disabilities

upheld or insofar as they are excluded from, or unable to gain access to, mainstream mechanisms for protection and redress.

Anti-discriminatory legislation and practice form an essential backdrop to the prevention of abuse. People with disabilities using the voice of the European Disability Forum (EDF) have clearly expressed the view that:

- many people with disabilities live in fear of violence;
- it is everyone's responsibility to challenge such violence and to challenge it at every level;
- responses are inadequate with inadequate access to public support or to mainstream routes for redress.

1.5. Aims of the report

The working group of the Council of Europe expects member states to consider a range of measures to assure the safety of disabled children and adults in their:

- homes;
- workplaces;
- service settings such as schools, day centres, residential homes, wider communities; and
- public places.

This report provides an illustrative framework within which member countries can consider:

- a workable definition of violence, abuse, mistreatment and neglect;
- case studies to show how these issues affect the lives of people with disabilities;
- an overview of research and sources of information on these issues;
- information to help professionals assess risk to people with disabilities;
- a brief account of how these issues are being addressed by member countries;

- examples of good practice in policy and service development; and
- an outline of the role of public and non-governmental organisations in response to issues of abuse in the lives of people with disabilities.

Case studies from different member states are included throughout the report to illustrate the range of situations under consideration and the particular issues which arise in different settings.

1.6. The structure of the report

The report is divided into six sections.

- Section 1 provides an introduction to the report, its scope, terminology and structure;
- Section 2 seeks to define what is meant by abuse and mistreatment and how it differs from more general problems of discrimination or from rightful use of force or detention;
- Section 3 provides an evaluation of recent research and summarizes what is known about the extent and causes of abuse. Difficulties in data gathering are noted in this section;
- Section 4 explores the legal framework and its contribution to protection;
- Section 5 sets out a range of preventative interventions and cites examples of good practice from different member countries;
- Section 6 sets out the working group's recommendations for action by member states highlighting the roles and responsibilities of governments and non-governmental social care agencies.

2. WHAT IS MEANT BY "ABUSE AND MISTREATMENT"?

2.1. Abuse: a process of definition

Abuse occurs when the integrity of any person is violated by another person who inflicts physical or psychological pain on them, or in situations where an individual's civil rights are breached, negated or ignored. The unequal power that accrues to adults in our society and particularly to adults in care-giving positions is an important factor in conceptualising abuse of children and of vulnerable adults (Brown & Turk 1992). Sexual and financial exploitation occurs where there is an absence of informed or un-coerced consent in a relationship or transaction including abuse of power or authority. Abuse may also be deemed to have occurred where a person's basic needs are not addressed in their family, community or society leading to cumulative or permanent harm, exclusion and/or serious deprivation.

Specific forms of abuse may also be crimes in member states, for example physical and sexual assaults, theft, deception and false imprisonment. Describing these acts as "abuse" may make them seem less serious or lead to them being dealt with through informal channels or in such a way that they attract less serious penalties or opprobrium than if their victims had been non-disabled children or adults (see Luckasson 1992; Williams & Evans 2000; Sobsey 1994).

Moreover abuse tends to have been conceptualised and/or prioritised differently by member states which have then taken the lead in addressing particular forms of abuse or mistreatment in different settings. For example, in the United Kingdom an initial focus on *sexual* abuse of people with intellectual disabilities took precedence over other (arguably more common) forms of physical abuse and coercion. The Flemish community in Belgium singled out pervasive forms of control and restraint as a priority. Furthermore, campaigns to highlight and remediate different forms of harm have tended to reflect different interests and have been routed through different channels. For example mental health service users have developed strong user-led networks to challenge statutory service provision whereas in other fields statutory service providers have taken on a "watchdog" role in relation to less regulated settings in private or voluntary service agencies or in family settings.

The working group has been very mindful of the gap between an "academic" definition of abuse and the complex realities that characterise the lives of people with disabilities and those who care for them. We include a number of brief case studies throughout this chapter that illustrate the issues under consideration and the sensitive professional judgments which need to be made when deciding whether intervention is warranted. The group has also been mindful of the inequity which exists between states across Europe and of the impact this has on disabled citizens of those countries.

Following Maslow (1943) we believe that needs which are negated can be conceptualised in a hierarchy. Rights to the most basic necessities of life such as adequate shelter, warmth, nutrition and health care are routinely denied in some countries particularly to people living in large institutions, while in other states more sophisticated demands for self-expression and actualisation are thwarted through discrimination and failure to observe civil liberties and civic status. This is not to say that equal citizenship rights and opportunities are any the less urgent or important but to act as a reminder that across Europe, some disabled people still live in conditions which jeopardise their lives as well as their livelihoods. Children may be born into such institutions with no separate assessment of their needs or proper chance of an ordinary childhood or family life.

2.1.1. Abuse by a range of people

The working group is concerned about abuse of both children and adults in a range of situations and settings. Disabled children and adults may be abused by people they know or by those who are responsible for their care; they may also be abused by their peers, by other young people or by other disabled service users whose abusing behaviour will need to be addressed by responsible authorities. They may also be the target of abuse by strangers, random violence or of hate crimes.

2.1.2. Abuse in a range of settings

Abuse takes place in a range of settings including disabled people's own homes, their family homes, foster or group living situations, ordinary community situations such as places of leisure or employment, schools, large scale institutions and day centres, hospitals and nursing homes. Upholding the rights of people with disabilities in prisons and other secure or restricted settings is of particular concern especially when people have mental illness or dual diagnoses (AEP 2000; Gabel 1996:53). Statutory and non-governmental agencies may have more or less access to, or influence in, these different situations. In some countries formal residential settings are regulated and regularly inspected and although this will not be enough to guarantee safety it provides an important route through which mistreatment can be challenged. Access to family settings may be more ad hoc for disabled adults than children, whose health and educational progress may be routinely monitored.

2.1.3. Institutional abuse

Abuse in institutional settings is regarded by many to be endemic and can take place against a pervasive culture of depersonalisation, lack of privacy, inactivity, inadequate food and heating, poorly trained and supervised staff and isolation from community activities. Programmes of hospital closure and de-institutionalisation have taken place in many countries with a preference for smaller community-based group living settings and this change is commended by the European Committee for the Prevention of Torture and Inhuman or Degrading Treatment of Punishment (CPT). Institutional abuse is being addressed in Spain through a programme of making institutions more open and accountable and through professional regulation. One of the objectives of the Spanish Action Plan for People with disabilities (Ministerio de Trabajo y Asuntos Sociales 1997) is also to promote a shift away from institutionalisation and support an active presence at home. A formal complaints procedure is described later in this report but despite new measures cases are often not formally notified because individuals fear reprisals or ostracism when they continue to depend on services provision. Italy has also had a major programme of replacing both psychiatric and mental disability hospitals in favour of community-based group residences.

Moving into communities is a necessary but not always a sufficient catalyst for good service provision. Service users still require skilled help and assistance to engage in activities of daily living and to sustain relationships. Staff in small homes may lack skills to engage people with profound or multiple difficulties or deal with difficult behaviour so that dangers/pressures escalate rapidly when people are living at close quarters. Smaller homes can also lead to professional isolation as only one or two staff may be on duty at a time. They may be less involved in professional networks or associations leading them to develop their own norms and idiosyncratic therapies or practices.

Smaller group homes or privately run nursing homes may also retain features of institutionalisation which lead to abuse even though they look more homely and are sited more locally. For example, they may still operate as closed systems with little contact from outside agencies and/or with inadequate accountability. Their hierarchies may reflect sexual or racial inequalities rather than knowledge or experience. Conditions of employment may be poor with staff working long hours, without unionisation or proper contracts, benefits or supervision. Recent research in the United Kingdom

(Hetherington 2000) suggested that the care sector was one of the worst for breaches in minimum wage legislation. One motivation for institutional closure was to break up vested interests and to remove barriers between "professionals" and service users. But in some cases deprofessionalisation has resulted in a casual and unregulated workforce. Care workers are often untrained and poorly paid, they may be subject to sexual harassment or bullying themselves and recycle this onto their clients. Moreover, community attitudes are not always supportive and people with disabilities may struggle to be accepted within their new neighbourhoods, sometimes facing blanket indifference or outright hostility.

2.2. Types of abuse

Abuse may be categorized at different levels. At a basic level it may take different forms including

- **physical violence,** including abusive use of corporal punishment, incarceration including being locked in one's home or not allowed out, over or mis-use of medication, medical experimentation or involvement in invasive research without consent;
- **sexual abuse and exploitation,** including rape, sexual aggression, indecent assaults, indecent exposure, involvement in pornography and prostitution;
- **psychological threats and harm** usually consisting of verbal abuse, intimidation, harassment, humiliation or threats of punishment or abandonment, emotional blackmail, arbitrariness, withholding adult status and infantilising disabled persons (see Département de la prévoyance sociale et des assurances 1997:12);
- **interventions which violate the integrity of the person,** including educational, therapeutic and behavioural programmes;
- **financial abuse,** fraud and theft of belongings, money or property;
- **neglect, abandonment and deprivation,** this may be physical or emotional and includes an often cumulative lack of

33

health care or negligent risk-taking, withdrawal of food or drink or other necessities of daily living including in the context of educational or behavioural programmes.

The European Disability Forum (EDF) (1999a:7) sets out a similar typology.

The Parliamentary Assembly of the Council of Europe (1998) has already made a series of recommendations relating to all children asking that member states incorporate protection of children against a range of abuses into their national legislation including:

- sexual abuse including paedophilia, exploitation and involvement in pornography, incest and prostitution;
- abuse, including abuse within the family;
- refusal of necessary care;
- inappropriate criminal proceedings;
- abusive sterilisation and violence and mutilation of girls.

Glaser and Bentovim (1979:567), pioneers in this field at the United Kingdom's leading children's hospital, have made a clear distinction between active and passive abuse, i.e. between "commission of injury" and "omission of care".

2.2.1. Physical punishment

In many European countries there is no outright prohibition of physical punishment although it has been banned in schools (for example in the United Kingdom it was banned in state schools in 1987 but maintained in private schools until 1999). In several states campaigns are underway to reduce the reliance on physical modes of punishment in child-rearing in all settings including in families. Member states are urged to move to an explicit ban as quickly as possible *particularly* for children with disabilities or special needs. This safeguard should be extended to all care homes and residential services for children and adults. Guidance may be needed to spell out the fact that disabled children are included in these directives, to highlight potentially abusive practices and to specify what methods of restraint (as opposed to punishment) are acceptable in different circumstances.

2.2.2. Inadequate health care

A number of concerns have been raised in relation to health care for people with disabilities. These include:

- discriminatory access to routine and preventative health care;
- rationing of interventions on account of disability rather than clinical need;
- a perceived readiness to accept euthanasia or non-intervention in cases of life threatening illness because of an individual's impairment;
- over, or inappropriate, use of sterilization and other intrusive or irreversible methods of contraception;
- neglect of personal hygiene to the extent that it presents real health hazards;
- over use of medication to control mood or suppress difficult behaviour;
- failure to respond to everyday illnesses and acute pain such as tooth-ache, period pains, ear-ache and stomach upsets (noted by Autism Europe).

One legacy of institutional models of care has been the tendency to medicalise every aspect of an individual's life but this does not equate to good medical care for people's illnesses as opposed to their impairments (Tilley 1998). Often where the person's impairment is the sole focus of medical intervention their ordinary health care needs are overlooked. Research suggests, for example, that cancer diagnoses are made very late for people with learning disabilities because symptoms are ignored or minimised (Read 1998). Recent research in the United Kingdom has highlighted inadequate and discriminatory access to screening and preventative health care for people with intellectual disabilities (Fovargue, Keywood & Flynn 1999) and differential access to cardiac surgery for children and adults with Down's Syndrome (Evans 2001).

The European Committee for the Prevention of Torture and Inhuman or Degrading Treatment or Punishment (CPT 1998) recommends a number of criteria for evaluating the health care provided to those who are involuntarily detained from which it is possible to infer a set of standards which apply equally to those who are voluntarily placed in residential or more informal care settings. These criteria were derived initially from the committee's work in prisons and are of particular importance in secure settings, for adults who do not have channels through which they can appeal and/or for those who lack capacity to evaluate their health care and/or seek alternative arrangements.

Key criteria include:

- access to an independent and appropriately qualified doctor;
- equivalence of care;
- respect for the patient's consent and confidentiality;
- access to preventative health care;
- professional independence and competence on the part of the doctor (European Committee for the Prevention of Torture and Inhuman or Degrading Treatment or Punishment (CPT)/Inf/(98)12).

Many disabled children and adults find themselves more informally "contained" or managed within their families, boarding schools, religious communities or residential settings. But the CPT's framework and the principle of equivalent access to health care provide a useful benchmark. Informality should not be taken as a signal that rights are being upheld. Judgments about the adequacy of care, nutrition and access to health care should always be made in relation to prevailing standards as these are applied to all citizens. Council of Europe Parliamentary Assembly Recommendation 1371 (1998) urges member states to pass legislation defining non-assistance as an offence in circumstances where a responsible person puts a child at risk by forgoing or refusing care. Where health care is provided within, and as part of, an overall institutional programme this principle of *equivalence* is particularly important.

Disability must not, of itself, be seen as a reason for refusing or rationing treatment, for withholding resuscitation or for withdrawing life-saving interventions. Where any such decisions are to be made these should be made transparently and on the basis of broad consultation. There should be provision for judicial review whenever life and death decisions, intrusive or irreversible treatments are to be authorised. Disabled or mentally ill persons need to be accorded specific and very visible protection and safeguards in relation to such interventions based on the principles of full and informed consent and/or advanced directives. This is particularly important in any countries that have legalised or quasi-legalised forms of euthanasia or physician-assisted suicide (Dyer 2001). Groups representing disabled people, with historical justification, express considerable fear about the potential for these to be applied in a discriminatory way, outside the intended parameters or as an alternative to properly resourced palliative care. Sterilisation raises similar fears and the need for comparable safeguards.

More routine health care decisions must be made proactively with, and where necessary on behalf of, people with disabilities. Individuals should not be left to make decisions which are outside their knowledge or competence. Services may lean towards non-intervention as part of a commitment to break with the past and to end intrusive institutional practices such as checking people's underwear to see if it is soiled several times a day or scrubbing people clean when ordinary washing is sufficient (cases raised by the Swiss delegation). These invasions of privacy were often justified on the basis of over-zealous attention to hygiene in services which allowed a medical model to dictate the tenor of everyday interactions. But at the other extreme, individuals should not be left to make decisions which are outside their knowledge or competence. Foubert (1998) cautions against neglect being justified on the grounds that it is the person's choice to avoid activity or refuse treatment when they are unable to take care of themselves.

> Jacques, a young disabled man who is autisitic lives in a small community-based residential setting during the week. He cannot wipe his own bottom after using the toilet. He cannot bring himself to look at his body or to touch himself and, in spite of extensive efforts to teach him, he cannot use toilet paper. Every Friday evening when he returns to his parents, they have to bath him and remove leftover faeces that have hardened on him during the week, sometimes to the extent that the only way to remove them is to cut his pubic hair. Staff at the residential unit claim their treatment of him is justified by their wish to encourage him to be independent and by their commitment not to invade his privacy.
>
> (Case study submitted by the Swiss delegation)

Simple rules cannot replace sensitive practice in situations such as this when principles seemingly contradict each other and the person's welfare may be compromised by non-intervention.

2.2.3. *Abuse by relatives or carers in the family home*

Families are legitimately involved in safeguarding their disabled family members and in managing their affairs but their involvement may be difficult to challenge and/or give rise to problems. Families may feel resentful if their actions are scrutinised or challenged after years of caring in which they have been unsupported by state or welfare agencies. On the other hand family members may not always know what is best, or be able to manage the care of their relative. Family members and onlookers may find it difficult to disentangle the interests of the disabled person from the family's own needs and entitlements. People with disabilities may not be well placed to challenge decisions made on their behalf by family members. Bringing such matters to the attention of the welfare agencies may also be difficult as outsiders may not know what is appropriate or who to contact. Intervening in such situations may then be carried out under different jurisdictions and with different assumptions and powers depending on whether the vulnerable person is a child or an adult.

> Hélène, a young woman with learning disabilities, lived with her parents, who did not seem to be caring for her properly. According to her neighbours, she was regularly "punished" by being left alone in the back yard, in the cold, without shoes and with little clothing. When her parents went out they forced her to stay in the yard until late at night. Eventually neighbours sent a collective letter to inform the relevant authorities of the situation.
>
> (Case study submitted by the Belgian delegation)

States vary in the extent they vest powers in parents to make decisions on behalf of a disabled child or adult, and in how far this is subject to scrutiny or judicial review. Major and irreversible interventions such as sterilisation of a mentally incapacitated child or adult need to be located in the courts to safeguard against excessive family control, especially around controversial issues such as independent living, sexuality, childbearing and risk-taking. The winner of an international film competition held in conjunction with the European Day of Disabled Persons 1999 conference addressed the distress caused to a young woman with cerebral palsy who had been pressured by her family into being sterilised against her wishes as a precursor to her marriage (Maroger 1999). A further French court case (in Sens, near Paris; Henley 2000a) referred to fourteen young women from a home for people with learning disabilities who had been sterilised without their knowledge over the last five years (see also Diederich 1998).

At a more mundane level there are many issues which give rise to potential conflicts of interest, for example absorption of welfare benefits into the family income, use of restraints or surveillance, the proper limits to household/domestic/farm work asked of the disabled family member and so forth. Adults with disabilities may be infantilised and denied their rights to an independent life of their own, to educational or social opportunities outside the home and to (consenting as opposed to exploitative) sexual relationships. The following case study illustrates this dynamic.

> Maria is a 25 year-old woman, diagnosed early on in life as schizophrenic. She is an only child and still lives at home with her elderly and very rigid parents. She has a degree in History, which

she obtained with great personal effort as well as help from her parents. However she had never worked, and the end of her studies was followed by a period where Maria's illness worsened. After two years which included intensive psychotherapy and psychiatric input, there was agreement between Maria, her psychologist and psychiatrist, that she was ready to hold down a job.

Her parents were apparently supportive of Maria's new life project but when a placement was found her parents reacted violently and forbade her to go, alleging that her new job was too far away and that it would be "dangerous" for her to use public transport where "anything could happen to her". The job was in a museum in the outskirts of town, and she had to catch two buses to get there. Even after being approached by the psychologist they were reluctant, stating that "in these conditions it was preferable that Maria should continue to stay at home and receive her disability subsidy" as this way she would "stay safe" and still have some money "to buy her little things".

(Case study from Portugal)

2.2.4. Abuse by, and in, service systems

The role is however often reversed when people are receiving services from state or welfare agencies. Parents and relatives may then find themselves critical of their relative's treatment and may not know how to challenge the "official" line or who will arbitrate if there is a genuine difference of opinion.

Michelle, a 42-year-old woman suffering from cystic fibrosis lived in residential care. The illness had left her with severe impairments and her family noticed that she had lost a lot of weight and complained when she was moved to a different wing in the home and seemed unhappy in this new group. Despite her family's requests, she was not allowed to return to her old wing and one day she was attacked by another patient and suffered a broken nose as a result. Her parents requested again that she be moved back to live with a less aggressive group as she could not defend herself. Nothing was done in response to this incident or to their requests. Moreover, Michelle continued to lose weight and the family subsequently learned that dietary recommendations they had been following for many years were no longer being adhered to: a doctor at the home later told them that this did not matter as the illness had already damaged her body so that the special diet was not necessary.

The family entered into a dispute with the establishment and took Michelle to live with them at home even though this created difficulties for them in relation to their jobs and caring responsibilities. Several weeks later the family received a letter from a Justice of the Peace informing them that an independent "administrator" had been appointed following a complaint by the medical services who regarded the family as posing a threat to their adult daughter.

(Case study submitted by the French-speaking community of Belgium)

Service users may avoid being caught in the middle in this way by organising their own networks and/or contacting independent advocates to take up their issues. People who use mental health services have been particularly concerned about abuses which are caused by the structure of services and abusive treatments, for example through unwarranted detention, inappropriate or enforced treatment, over-medication, use of Electro Convulsive Therapy (ECT) and loss of civil liberties. Concern has also been voiced by the European Committee for the Prevention of Torture and Inhuman or Degrading Treatment or Punishment (CPT), and by user groups, about abuse of one service user by another as a result of inappropriate placements (as in Michelle's case cited above), too few staff and inadequate training. Women have campaigned for separate spaces in asylums and day services as one safeguard against sexual harassment and violence by other service users.

The submission of the Flemish community in Belgium also notes the dual meanings of "institutionalised" as both violence which occurs in institutions and violence which is institutionalised in that it is legitimised by law. State-condoned violence against people with disabilities has and may still include:

• incarceration without due process or avenues for appeal or review;

41

- enforced sterilisation or compulsory abortions when pregnant;
- not being allowed to marry or engage in sexual relationships, including gay or lesbian relationships;
- not being given assistance to bring up children; or having those children removed without formal assessment or care planning;
- inappropriate groupings and lack of choice about whom to live with or options to leave group settings in which violence is a daily occurrence highlighted in a number of case studies submitted to the working group;
- being forced to observe religious rules which are not of their choosing because religious organisations are their only source of practical assistance and accommodation; or conversely being hindered from following their religion when it is of their choosing for example when people with disabilities from ethnic minorities are placed in congregate residential settings;
- exclusion from work places and from public places on account of non-accessible public buildings and public transport.

Rules may be in force in institutions which are not in accordance with international law. For example, there may be discrimination on grounds of sexual orientation in the way institutions "allow" relationships between patients; rights to privacy, to receive mail or make telephone calls may be breached routinely; people may be informally (i.e. without due process or independent scrutiny) detained or restrained. Even where these practices are not explicitly condoned by member states they may still occur on a widespread basis.

Other so-called "professional" practices may be accepted as legitimate without challenge in some member states including:

- solitary confinement;
- control and restraint;
- medical castration;

- over-reliance on sedation as a means of control;

- punishment or deprivation as part of a behavioural programme;

- unmodified Electro Convulsive Therapy (ECT) (that is without use of anaesthesia).

Legal safeguards around these practices are dealt with in more detail in chapter 4.

Services have to provide policies and training to support staff in *how* to respond positively to difficult behaviour or situations. Guidance which merely articulates a set of ideals, without detailed instructions about how to put values into practice, may drive a wedge between direct care staff and their managers who "officially" distance themselves from daily pressures and dilemmas while tacitly acknowledging that they have no alternative to offer.

Coercive treatment was the focus of the following case study.

> Paul was one of three children with a learning disability as well as disturbed behaviour due to mental health problems. As a teenager he attended a boarding school but spent weekends at home. When he became an adult his behaviour grew more difficult to manage and he was placed in a psychiatric hospital surrounded by other people with behaviour problems. He received little care and his condition worsened. He was finally transferred to a specialist unit, as a result of his parents' campaigning, where he received individualised care in a more positive environment. He made progress, there were positive changes and his parents were happy. However the hospital was 200 kllometres from their home and since they were elderly they had very little contact with their son. As he got older, the hospital staff decided to treat Paul with electro-convulsive therapy as he had been displaying bouts of aggression. They contacted the parents for their opinion and went ahead with the family's consent. The staff believed that this was the only way of controlling his behaviour. The treatment was stopped after one month: the effects had been disastrous and his condition had worsened.
>
> (Case study submitted by a Belgian NGO)

Electro Convulsive Therapy (ECT) is a controversial treatment and one whose efficacy is disputed. The NGO who submitted this case study commented that:

"some scientists are reintroducing these terrifying methods, which were quite rightly discarded for several decades. Their intentions are perhaps commendable but the means are inappropriate. The effects of treatment are far worse than the illness..."

Strong safeguards and a sound evidence base are needed to ensure that disputed treatments are not administered inappropriately or without proper consent. In this case the parents were not in a position to act as advocates for their son or to substitute their consent instead of his. People with behaviour problems and dual diagnoses are particularly at risk of such interventions at the hands of medical or other professional authorities and their families may not be in a position to advocate strongly for alternatives.

The same applies to participation in research projects, especially those which include intrusive interventions and/or which carry some risk. Particular concern should be paid to people who cannot themselves give valid consent or who may be susceptible to pressure from those in authority. The working group expresses its particular concern about such participtation when the research is not directly in the participants' own interest. Exceptions to this should be decided transparently by publicly accountable ethical committees and/or be subject to appeal.

2.3. Some underlying factors

2.3.1. Financial abuse and the structure of benefits

Financial abuse is a problem in itself but member states, NGO's and user groups are also concerned about how structural problems in the benefits system as well as inadequate levels of benefit limit the possibilities for people with disabilities to live a life of their choice, to have a range of adult relationships and/or to escape violence.

44

Financial arrangements may set up unhelpful contingencies which provide a backdrop to abusive situations. A number of issues were raised in and by case studies including:

- public finance arrangements which are weighted towards institutional care rather than community-based alternatives, leaving individuals in a situation where they can only get full support if they agree to live in an institution and putting pressure on relatives to "choose" this kind of care;

- means tested benefits which penalise the person and/or their partner or parents if they work to earn a wage which is above the poverty line;

- benefits which allow assets to be taken as future payment for needed services: this sets up a situation in which relatives who might eventually be beneficiaries of the person's estate have a conflict of interest in deciding whether or not to seek help when caring becomes too arduous for them;

- arrangements which attract benefits to the individual or to their relative/carer but which do not include any scrutiny to ensure that the standard of care reflects the amount granted: this allows a situation to develop in which an unscrupulous relative might gain financially from providing inadequate care;

- benefits which assume that a partner or relative will assume complete financial responsibility for the disabled person: this creates dependence and/or resentment and makes it very difficult for the disabled person to leave if they wish or if they need to escape violence or mistreatment;

- payments which allow individuals no choice over where they access help which is paid for out of their benefits (unlike models of independent living using direct payments in which the disabled person and/or their relatives are able to employ their own carers).

The following case study illustrates some of these problems:

Ms N. is a woman of 53 who contracted poliomyelitis at the age of 16 and spent many years on a ventilator in a large hospital, much of it in a ward for people with terminal illnesses. During her time there she became very skilled as an informal social worker and

45

studied for a degree and professional qualification in psychology. She met and married a man through a friend and left hospital to live with him in her late 20s. Ms N. has shown remarkable fortitude and generosity throughout her life, at one time establishing a communal residence for other people with disabilities and a foundation to support people with disabilities in former eastern bloc countries. She needs assistance for 12 hours a day which is very expensive and her benefits do not cover this amount. The standard health insurance will pay for one hour's care: her husband has to work long hours to cover the additional cost with variable donations from charitable individuals. If she were re-admitted to residential care it would cost the authorities considerably more. Ms N. is becoming increasingly despondent: stress is upsetting her family and the people who live in the residential community she founded. Each month there is a shortage of money. Despite begging letters for help, savings have been used up and her whole life is overshadowed by the possibility that she will have to endure once again the state of dependence and despair she experienced in hospital.

(Case study submitted by the Swiss delegation)

This example shows how the social insurance system itself, when organised in a particular manner, can exercise a form of "structural violence" by significantly limiting the choices the people with disabilities may make as for their way of life. On the one hand, a person in need of care and professional guidance is dependent on the assistance of specialised service providers who are not able to satisfy all the needs of the disabled person. For example, the person concerned cannot choose his or her carer, nor the time when the care is received (such as help for lying down on the bed). On the other hand, the insurance provision for the care and professional guidance (e.g. health care insurance and disability pension) only cover a fraction of the expenses incurred if the disabled person lives in her or his own home. The expenses are only covered in full when the person lives in an institution. As a result, many people with disabilities have no other option but to enter an institution simply on financial grounds.

Providing adequate benefits does however create its own dynamics. The French-speaking community of Belgium submitted the following case study:

> Denise who has severe learning disabilities had been living in res-
> idential care for twenty years. Her brother, Albert, who was also
> disabled, was also living there. Their brothers and sisters did not
> play any part in their care until after Albert's death when they
> reappeared and, discovering that their sister was in receipt of
> social security benefits, one of the sisters who was experiencing
> financial difficulties herself offered to take Denise out of the home
> and care for her at home. Denise was very happy to see her
> unknown but seemingly kind sister again and was not in any posi-
> tion to weigh up her offer or to appreciate her ulterior motives.

Other delegates questioned the adequacy of arrangements for
the administration of financial matters on behalf of people
unable to make their own decisions and on the safeguards
and scrutiny within the system in these situations. A case submitted by the Belgian delegation concerned a family with
three intellectually disabled siblings as a result of Fragile X
syndrome whose uncle was appointed their legal guardian on
the death of their parents. This uncle (the father's brother) was
supposed to operate under the supervision of another uncle
(the mother's brother).

> The legal guardian kept the benefit payments, withdrew money
> from the bank accounts of the young people with learning disabili-
> ties and even succeeded in selling a flat that one of them had inher-
> ited. Delayed payments to the care home gave rise to suspicion and
> the guardian's son approached the parents association partly to
> "whistle-blow" and partly to distance himself from any wrong-
> doing. The parents association contacted a Justice of the Peace who
> took action but the remedies available would have meant compen-
> sation being sought over a prolonged period from this already aged
> uncle and the disabled siblings would never recover their assets.

In this country's legal system the supervision of guardians
was left to relatives and once misappropriation of funds had
taken place the law proved virtually unenforceable.

2.3.2. Abusive ideologies

Other important issues also colour the debate – as the
European Disability Forum (1999a:12) makes clear:

> "Violence can take not only active but also passive forms such as
> euthanasia and eugenics, resulting in particular in compulsory

47

> *sterilisation, sexual segregation and the development of biotechnology and prenatal diagnosis."*

Some social commentators (for example Wolfensberger 1987) have argued that there is a tendency towards and alliance with death expressed through a *"hidden policy of genocidal destruction of certain of [society's] rejected and unwanted classes"* in modern societies which renders all people with disabilities vulnerable. While the development of bio-technology and pre-natal diagnosis might not in itself be considered abusive, it is considered a potential threat by many people with disabilities and their organisations because it is seen to rest on the untenable assumption that the quality of life of people with disabilities is inevitably poorer than that of non-disabled people. The "expressivity" argument is that the practice of pre-natal screening and selective abortion sends out powerful signals to disabled people that society does not value them or consider their lives to be worth living (Parens & Asch 2000; Ward 2001). People with disabilities fear, with historical justification, that if held in its most extreme forms, this mindset may lead to discriminatory end-of-life decisions, increased uptake of selective abortion of handicapped foetuses, rationing of health care and discriminatory treatment of disabled persons.

People with disabilities and their organisations clearly interpret these developments as contributing to a set of values which are hostile to them and which encourage lack of respect for the worth of their lives. At street level these attitudes are expressed through harassment and intimidation in public places, for example people shouting at a disabled person "You should not have been born!" or threatening to gas them. The isolation of people with disabilities is exacerbated when they are afraid to go out or to enter public places and spaces for fear of verbal or physical harassment.

2.4. Doubly disadvantaged groups

2.4.1. Abuse of people from ethnic minorities

Abuse of disabled children and adults also takes place against the backdrop of broader, and often multiple, forms of oppression, exploitation, social injustice and conflict. People with disabilities from ethnic minorities are doubly disadvantaged in their dealings with social and welfare institutions and in their vulnerability to racially motivated abuse and discrimination. These "extra" disadvantages are not separate entitites, running in parallel, but act as multipliers of difficulty and create a unique identity for disabled individuals who may be resisting hostile attitudes to disability within their own communities at the same time as they are struggling with the effects of social and economic discrimination due to racism from the dominant community (Stewart 1993).

People with disabilities and their relatives/carers from ethnic minorities may also be disadvantaged in not being able to access social care services equitably. A study of ethnic minority carers of older people in the United Kingdom (Netto 1998) showed that they tended to be younger and more isolated than white carers, with half not able to speak the predominant language, three-quarters were women many of whom also cared for children; they cared over a longer period, had less help from other members of the family and had no provision for time–off to meet their own needs. Also Netto (1998: 223) points out that they often do not identify themselves as "carers" and hence did not articulate their entitlement to support services:

> *"this is hardly surprising, as ...?carers' is a socio-political construct whose currency is much more closely tied into rights to practical support than to the feelings and relationships which motivate care-giving, the word has no equivalent in any of the minority ethnic languages."*

Mainstream services are frequently provided in ways which fail to recognise or accommodate religious or cultural differences: they may not provide food which respects religious or dietary needs, carers of the same sex to provide personal care or single sex services where these would be preferred. At the same time agencies and workers may fail to engage in a proper debate with people from minority cultures for example about stigmatising and unscientific beliefs about disability, appropriate discipline or punishment of children or about treatment of women which breaches civil liberties as guaranteed under the European Convention on Human Rights. Some campaigning organisations working with people with disabilities from ethnic minorities have begun to raise issues about consent and rights within arranged marriages.

The working group has been particularly mindful of the position of people with disabilities in countries affected by war and of the particular pressures on people with disabilities who have been forced to become refugees (currently subject of research in the United Kingdom being carried out at the Social Policy Unit at the University of York). Not only do these conflicts lead to increased levels of trauma-related physical and mental disability, sometimes made worse by lack of subsequent medical assistance, but individuals have to come to terms with such events against a backdrop of economic and social disruption which acts as a barrier to medical and social rehabilitation. Countries, which have recently been at the centre of conflict, are also trying to offer aid to refugees. Slovenia is currently giving asylum to 2796 persons from Bosnia and Herzegovina. According to official statistics, at least 42 of them are disabled. Some of these refugees have already been living in Slovenia for eight years and many have no place to return to. Data is not available about the level of physical or mental disability experienced by people with disabilities in war-torn countries or about whether other people with disabilities had been unable to escape their former homes when the conflict was at its height.

Attitudes to people with disabilities in war-time become polarised and contradictory. At the time, the sacrifice of someone who becomes disabled for their homeland is highly valued. This makes people feel that they have sacrificed for their country the most that they had and that after the war they should acquire more rights than other citizens. But when the war is over and they want to include themselves in normal life they are not accepted.

Individuals come to comprehend their sacrifice as having no sense at all and resent the restricted status they are accorded. Under-age soldiers are an especially tragic group: not only because of the wounds to their bodies but because as youngsters they do not comprehend and cope easily with death. Participation in the war has caused heavy, if not irreparable, consequences to their souls, their personalities, their feelings and behaviour which later on, in time of peace, hinders their return to everyday life, prevents them from creating their own families and establishing solid relationships with other people. Their problems are exacerbated by the structure of disability benefits which preclude employment possibilities. They want to recreate their lives and develop their potential and not to be only the receivers of disability allowances.

(Extract from Slovenia's submission to the working group).

People with disabilities in war-torn countries face a very particular struggle to achieve full citizenship. They consider themselves to have "earned" an entitlement to proper benefits and service provision given that they have sacrificed more than others. And they subsequently feel more disillusioned than others when they find themselves forgotten as memories of the struggle recede or when they find themselves facing all the barriers which disabled people face in other countries and situations. These disadvantages extend to those who seek refuge or asylum in other countries (Roberts 2000; Hermansson, Hornquist & Timpka 1996; AEP 2000) who may also fall between several stools when it comes to seeking a support community. Roberts (2000: 944) argues that the disability movement has yet to address the diversity of its membership and that "awareness of people with disabilities with the most complex identities is still lacking". She (2000: 944) asserts that:

"disabled refugees and asylum seekers, whose identities encompass, (at the very least), those of refugees, people with disabilities and minority ethnic groups, remain lost, because they are not recognised by either the refugee community (because of their impairments) or by the disability movement (because of their immigration status). Yet, disabled refugees and asylum seekers probably constitute one of the most disadvantaged groups within our society precisely because of their simultaneous experience of the economic and social disadvantages encountered by [these groups]."

51

2.4.2 Abuse of women and girls

Disabled girls and women share the disadvantages of all girls and women and are disproportionately victims of sexual violence and sexual harassment (Sorheim 1998). A comparable document on the prevention of violence against women identifies three layers or sites of gender-based oppression to which all disabled women (and some men, for example gay men or black men) may be especially vulnerable, that is physical, sexual and psychological violence occurring both in the context of the family and the wider community. The former includes battering, child abuse, marital rape and exploitation of girls and women through excessive demands on them to perform tasks such as unpaid care of children or elders, housework, farm work or industrial work at home. Sexual abuse in the community may take the form of sexual harassment and intimidation at work, trafficking in women and enforced prostitution. Women are also subjected to intrusive treatments and breaches of human rights in respect of issues such as compulsory abortion or sterilisation. Work is also a site of exploitation of women and girls in low paid or dangerous employment. Domestic workers face both private and public risks where their workplace is also a potential site of domestic violence.

Tilley (1998: 89) also points out how women with disabilities are doubly affected by stereotypes relating to disability and gender so that as women they are *"represented ... as victims, stereotypes of dependence which reinforces the 'sick' role often ascribed to people with disabilities"* while their disability sees them consigned to the status of *"seconds"* in a capitalist culture which values women predominantly for their appearance and as commodities. Intellectual disability or mental illness may also play into sexualised caricatures that portray women as unable to control their sexual impulses. The working group supports the recommendations set out in Council of Europe Parliamentary Assembly Recommendation 1450 (2000) including those which condemn domestic violence, forced marriage, genital mutilation, prostitution and trafficking in women and urges governments and NGOs to acknowledge that these breaches of human rights are also visited on women with disabilities who may have even fewer avenues for leaving violent relationships, entering refuges or seeking appropriate redress. Hendey and Pascall (1998:426) for example, drew attention to the risks inherent in the situation of disabled women who use direct payments to organise and manage their own personal assistants and who may find themselves in situations characterised by *"a painful lack of means to escape"*.

2.5. Making sensitive judgments

2.5.1. Thresholds

The working group has been mindful of the need for sensitivity in making balanced judgments which uphold disabled people's rights without unnecessarily interfering in the way they live their lives, or in the arrangements and relationships which emerge in families caring for a disabled person or in properly run establishments providing such care. In addition, member states may be under considerable economic pressures or subject to political and economic instability with multiple interest groups to satisfy and needs to prioritise.

Each country and agency will need to determine where the threshold lies in deciding when abuse reaches a sufficiently serious or persistent level to warrant an outside challenge. Such challenges may be made via different routes, for example through regulation of service provision, social work with individual families, action by user groups, criminal proceedings or legal action.

2.5.2. Respecting choice and consent

People with disabilities may not always wish to take action against those who harm them nor want outside authorities to do so on their behalf. The state has a clear responsibility to intervene when children are at risk but a more ambivalent role in relation to disabled adults. The twin concepts of capacity and informed consent are crucial to these judgments.

53

Where people are not able to make their own decisions, sexual acts and financial transactions may be construed as abusive and the state is the only body with a remit to step in and act for their protection. But a disabled person who usually acts autonomously may also be so undermined by violence or intimidation that intervention is necessary even if it is initially refused by them: this has parallels for other victims of serious crime. On the other hand people who are able to exercise their autonomy may from time to time enter into less than ideal relationships or put up with services that do not meet all of their needs but accept these as drawbacks in an otherwise acceptable situation. Many choices are made pragmatically between "the lesser of two evils", and it will be up to responsible agencies to draw a line for example in situations where only one option is offered or where choices are invalidated by threats, force or deliberate exploitation.

The legal principles used to determine capacity and consent are set out in Chapter 4. This chapter is concerned primarily with definition but these issues are illustrated in the following case studies in which an assessment of the person's capacity is the key to whether the relationship is, or is not, abusive. These situations all involved sexual relationships but similar issues arise in discriminating acceptable from exploitative financial transactions.

In the first case a 12 year-old-boy receiving special education at a boarding school had been abused by a teacher who was supposedly giving the child extra tuition in arithmetic. The child's behaviour changed and he hesitantly told his parents what was happening. The teacher had reached orgasm by kissing and touching the child's genitalia. The parents tried to get the head-teacher, the police and the medical centre to take action but they all deferred. Eventually a court case led the teacher to admit his paedophile tendencies and that he had used his profession to gain access to children. He was given a heavy sentence by the court. The child suffered long-term psychological harm as a result of this experience.

(Case submitted by the Swiss delegation from an NGO)

In this case there was no debate about the child having given valid consent – the child was under-age and therefore legally and morally unable to consent to sex with any adult, let alone an adult in a position of authority over him. This principle would still apply even if the young person had seemed willing to comply with the teacher's actions. A disabled adult who lacked the ability to make her or his own decisions would also be unable to consent to a relationship of this kind. A similar case was submitted by the Flemish community in Belgium concerning a young person with disabilities who was abused by a monk who was a department head at the residential home in which he lived. Even if the young person had been over the age of consent the power which this man exerted was so disproportionate that the act was clearly abusive.

This "abuse of trust" principle is carried over into certain therapeutic and professional relationships involving adults, such as counselling, health-related or pastoral care. In these relationships even when they involve people who are not vulnerable as a result of physical or mental disability, clients put themselves at risk. The relationship is unequal in that one person's time is being paid for by the other, in the expectation that the professional will meet the needs of their client and not seek to meet their own sexual or emotional needs in breach of this understanding.

Another issue raised by this case is the need for agreed mechanisms for sharing information which would usually be kept confidential and governed by data protection legislation. In a case like this the confidentiality principle would be overridden on account of the risk of significant harm occurring or continuing if information were not disclosed across agency/professional boundaries.

But consent issues are not always as clear-cut. A further case from the Swiss delegation highlighted confusion about the principles on which intervention may be based.

This situation concerned a woman with mild learning disabilities and limited communication skills who lived in a mixed institution. She became involved with two men at the same time and each

55

knew about the other. She managed to switch between the two but several members of the educational staff disapproved of her behaviour. In the name of fidelity as a criterion, the staff told the woman that she must choose between the two men which she refused to do. The staff then decided that she should stop seeing both of the men and took steps to prevent any further contact between them.

In this case the issue is more one of failing to support and uphold the young woman's right to choose how she conducts her relationships than of protection from harm, since these relationships were both of her choosing. A similar case from the United Kingdom reported in Brown and Thompson (1997) concerned two men who had a consenting gay relationship which was disapproved of in their residential home – a home run by a Christian charity. But in placing the men in this home the social services department should have taken their sexuality into account and by prohibiting their sexual relationship the service provider failed to respect their right to a lifestyle of their choosing.

Meanwhile another case submitted by the Swiss delegation which also concerned a young woman living in a mixed institution illustrated the opposite side of the coin where choice was being accepted at face value without enough consideration of the power dynamics which were influencing the situation.

This young woman had been put on a long-acting contraceptive injection ostensibly as a result of menstrual problems. Staff took this as a signal that they need not supervise her too closely even though she was a rather non-assertive person and was not well informed about sexual matters. No-one noticed or took the trouble to find out that this woman was intimidated by one of the men who had befriended her. When she asked him to leave after he had visited her in her room he grunted angrily and eventually she became nervous of all the men in the institution.

In this situation lack of sex education and avenues for confiding in others seriously failed this woman. The regime erred on the side of being permissive without equipping the residents to protect themselves or to be vigilant about consequences other than pregnancy.

Informed consent is a critical issue in defining abuse and service providers have to tread a careful line between testing out people's choices and upholding the rights of those who legitimately opt for an unconventional lifestyle. Decisions have to be made which take into account the wishes of the more vulnerable person and the intentions and motivation of the more powerful and perhaps potential abuser. Where either are stark a decision will be relatively clear but in those cases where a relationship of choice for one person is one of exploitation for the other, a balanced judgment has to be arrived at.

2.5.3. Assessing seriousness

Brown and Stein (1998) identified a set of criteria to be considered when trying to ascertain the threshold at which an incident or relationship demands more formal intervention or a disclosure of information, which would usually have been kept confidential, beyond a professional or agency boundary. Factors to take into account include (adapted from AIMS project 1998):

- the vulnerability of the victim, for example their frailty, the extent of their impairments, cognitive or communication difficulties;

- how extensive the abusive act(s) have been, for example French criminal law defines physical violence to be a serious offence when it results in at least 8 days' sick leave for the victim and English legislation speaks of "significant harm";

- whether the abuse has been a single incident or part of a long-standing pattern or relationship;

- what impact the abuse has had on the vulnerable person;

- whether others in the family or setting have been badly affected by, or drawn into, the abuse;

- the intent of the abuser and a judgment about whether the abuse was intended or inadvertent, arising out of stress or ignorance; and whether the abuser had set out to exploit this individual by targeting them specifically on account of their perceived disabilities. A view will need to be taken about whether the abuse was passive or active, wilful or accidental;

- the authority of the abuser and the extent to which they abused a "position of trust" for example where abuse is perpetrated by someone with standing in the community such as a priest, teacher, doctor, nurse, social worker;

- whether the abuse was such that it constituted a criminal offence;

- if there is a risk of repeated abuse from this abuser to this victim: for example sexual crime against either children or adults is more likely to be part of a pattern of serial offending rather than a one-off lapse of good character;

- what risk there is that this abuser or this setting will cause harm to other children or vulnerable adults?

The risk of "significant harm" marks the watershed in such an assessment. A judgment about seriousness inevitably takes place against the background of prevailing cultural and economic conditions especially when evaluating standards of care deemed adequate in each country and setting. It may be that a model of individual abuse is not the most effective way of achieving change if abusive practice or neglect permeates a whole service system or if people with disabilities are disproportionately affected by more widespread forms of poverty and deprivation.

2.6. Summary

As the French and Norwegian delegations note:

> "the difficulty of this exercise is to properly locate the problem at the right distance between two poles, first a reductive definition of violence ... which would obscure the reality of the phenomenon and second the exaggerated extension of the concept, which would dilute its specificity through including, much wider problems ... "

58

With this in mind, the working group is concerned about this broad range of sources and types of harm to people with disabilities including:

- seriously inadequate care and attention to basic needs including nutrition, health care and access to educational and social opportunities;

- individual acts of cruelty or sexual aggression by persons who are in the role of care givers;

- breaches of civil liberties such as incarceration without due process, "enforced cohabitation" in group homes or institutions, prohibition of sexual relationships or marriage, lack of privacy or intrusion into or interruption of mail or telephone calls or visits, in institutional or family settings and/ or continued isolation from sources of support or advocacy;

- acts of bullying or random violence within community settings, some of which may represent more extreme forms of generally held prejudice against people with disabilities or, of greater concern, global ideologies which are inimical to disabled persons;

- practice by individual staff which falls well outside, or below, accepted professional norms;

- abuses by other service users within service settings where attention has not been paid to safe groupings or sufficient supervision to ensure safe placements;

- authorised treatments and interventions which are not in the person's best interests and/or which rest on an inaccurate or incomplete understanding of their condition and needs, for example punitive responses to challenging behaviour, seclusion, unconsented ECT, or aversive behavioural programmes.

In summary, abuse is:

Any act, or failure to act, which results in a significant breach of a vulnerable person's human rights, civil liberties, bodily integrity, dignity or general well-being, whether intended or inadvertent, including sexual relationships or financial transactions to which the person has not or cannot validly consent, or which are deliberately exploitative.

Abuse may be perpetrated by any person (including by other people with disabilities) but it is of special concern when it takes place within a relationship of trust characterised by powerful positions based on:

- legal, professional or authority status,
- unequal physical, economic or social power,
- responsibility for the person's day-to-day care,
- and/or inequalities of gender, race, religion or sexual orientation.

It may arise out of individual cruelty, inadequate service provision or society's indifference.

It requires a proportional response one which does not cut across valid choices made by individuals with disabilities but one which does recognise vulnerability and exploitation.

Table 1: Elements of definition

Which people with disabilities are covered?

Children and adults with:

- physical, sensory and intellectual impairments;
- mental illness;
- autism;
- chronic illness.

What types of harm?

- physical;
- sexual;
- psychological;
- financial;
- neglect.

Who is the abuser?

All persons including:

- family members;
- other people with disabilities;
- paid staff and volunteers;
- influential people such as church leaders or teachers;
- neighbours;
- members of the public;
- strangers;
- professions such as in health care or the criminal justice system and including licensed therapists and social care staff;
- service providers;
- statutory agencies: both local and national authorities and governments.

In what settings?

All settings including:

- disabled people's own homes;
- family homes;
- residential settings, including boarding out and foster placements;
- schools;
- work places and day centres;
- health care settings;
- institutions, including secure settings and prisons;
- leisure facilities;
- public places, parks, transport, shops.

What is the threshold for reporting and action?

Assessment of seriousness depends on:

- wider cultural and economic norms;
- nature, frequency and extent of harm;
- if act constitutes a criminal offence;
- frailty of person;
- intent and perceived dangerousness of abuser;
- risk of repeated harm to individual;
- risk of harm to other disabled children or adults.

3. AWARENESS AND RESEARCH

These issues in definition and judgment spill over into research making it difficult to design studies and compare findings. Researchers often set out to answer clear-cut questions only to find themselves having to interpret ambiguous findings and read between the lines of their data to see the whole picture. Even where rigorous research designs are used (for example those incorporating matched control groups), under-reporting and inconsistent recording make comparisons difficult (Westcott 1991). There is however a growing literature on the abuse of children and adults with disabilities from which the following summary is drawn.

3.1. Methodological issues

In order to read this body of work it is important to appreciate why the research is not yielding definitive answers. Complex ethical and methodological issues have to be taken into account in the design and interpretation of studies:

- Labelling an act or relationship abusive is necessarily a matter of judgment and negotiation;

- Identification relies on personal, professional and organisational skills: abuse often takes place behind closed doors and abusers may take steps to pressurise those they have harmed into keeping secrets. A victim's distress, a perpetrator's lack of boundaries, reports of witnesses, or disclosure by any of the parties involved can easily be missed or ignored;

- People who have communication difficulties and/or are not accorded credibility may not have their complaints taken seriously and are therefore more likely to be overlooked in reports of abuse when compared with non-disabled people;

• Studies may rely on records or retrospective reports, the recall of which is in itself a test of organisational competency and stability;

• Studies are often not comparing like with like: a unit or case may refer to an act, a relationship, a person or a regime – single incidents may be noted alongside repeated abuses which have taken place within a longstanding exploitative relationship. Even where care is taken in definition, an act as it is reported may be the first which has occurred in this context or merely the one which triggered disclosure;

• Relatively minor incidents may be analysed alongside major traumatic events for those experiencing them;

• Disabled children and adults may be invisible within "mainstream" statistics for example those collated on child protection interventions or about crime involving the general population: this is the case across member states and was identified as an issue by the Italian delegation.

Many studies are necessarily based on samples of *reported* cases, documenting referrals to helping agencies which are contingent on that agency's reputation, approach and resources. Biases are inevitable in such data and interpretation is open to many questions: for example a raised rate of reporting may indicate a service which is more sensitive to the possibility of abuse and more open to hearing and taking note of allegations or disclosures. An agency which documents abuse in service settings but not in families does not demonstrate that abuse in families does not exist but that their own mechanisms for gaining entry to families and/or giving people with disabilities routes for disclosure beyond their family networks may be inadequate. In some countries a referral to statutory agencies is perceived as potentially stigmatising which in turn may lead to fewer reports of abuse. Paradoxically high rates of reporting may be a sign of good services not of abusive ones.

Meanwhile more informal NGO type agencies such as help lines, refuges or drop in centres will often draw on a diverse, and difficult to define, population. They may receive reports from anonymous sources and be unable to cross-check for double counts or for reports which have also been filed with other agencies in their areas. Nevertheless, specialist services, can provide valuable information about those cases which do come to their attention and they should be assisted in carrying out practice based research. The reliability of such research is best assured by mechanisms such as "triangulation" that is the consideration of data gathered from different perspectives and samples. In this sense abuse research has more in common with service evaluation or qualitative research studies than with more orthodox epidemiological studies.

A recent Slovenian survey carried out as part of the preparation of this report canvassed returns from NGO's serving people who are victims of violence: a help line for women and children responding to at least 3000 persons each year report that each month they provide counselling to someone receiving psychiatric treatment and that of 30 women attending a self-help group two were physically disabled. In 2000, Slovenia offered five shelters to victims of violence and six maternal homes, which provide room and board, legal representation, assistance in the handling of personal matters, participation in self-help groups and preparation for the future. However, these institutions are not adapted to persons using wheelchairs, although the staff are ready to adjust to such persons and meet them outside the institution. People with disabilities often use the available telephone and psychosocial counselling services and participate in self-help groups.

There has also been a bias towards studies of incidence and prevalence and away from work on the long-term consequences of abuse or the efficacy of therapeutic and service interventions. Exceptions include the Centre for young victims of abuse in Milan which takes care of the problems of both children and families (eg lack of attention, physical and sexual abuse) and also conducts research into specialised intervention programmes; as well as the United Kingdom programmes for young sex offenders and for sex offenders with learning disabilities which have been rigorously evaluated (see Vizard, Monk & Misch 1995; Vizard *et al.* 1996; Murphy 1997). Other models of service delivery and responses to abuse have been less well documented. There are also important links to be made across the usual boundaries of academic specialism. Disabled children are disproportionately affected by economic deprivation. Westcott and Jones (1999) commented that the earlier studies around children with disabilities focused on the presence of impairments in samples of abused children rather than the experience of abuse in the lives of disabled children, thereby missing a wealth of information. The link between the two fields of study has been signalled for many years (see, for example, Glaser & Bentovim 1979; Valentine 1990; Verdugo, Bermejo & Fuertes 1995) as abuse undoubtedly *causes* some impairments while impairment renders some individuals more vulnerable to abuse and/or makes disclosure more difficult. Few researchers work across these areas of specialism. Jaudes and Diamond (1985) explored the incidence of impairment as a consequence of child abuse; Kaplan *et al.* (1998) demonstrated an association between adolescent physical abuse and psychiatric disorders; Rose, Peabody and Stratigeas (1991) emphasised abuse as a precursor of adult mental ill health albeit one which is often glossed over in routine psychiatric assessments. Cohen and Warren (1990:254) noted that:

> *"The literature is replete with evidence that children who are abused or neglected are at greater risk of becoming emotionally disturbed, language impaired, mentally retarded, and/or physically disabled, while children with disabilities may be at greater risk of abuse and neglect."*

But the problem of working across professional disciplines, agencies and systems has fragmented the knowledge base which does exist.

For a "case" to be reported a number of hurdles have to be crossed. Abuse is essentially secret and some perpetrators put considerable effort into "grooming" a vulnerable person and creating an intimidating situation which enforces their secrecy. Where regimes are at fault senior managers may seek to suppress complaints or whistle-blowing. Research studies based on survey data, however thoroughly prepared and carried out, are likely to miss important data. If a survey relies on retrospective returns it becomes a test of administrative systems as well as of initial alertness and sensitivity to the abuse. In a study carried out using this methodology Brown, Stein and Turk (1995) found that one third of cases were forgotten within one year and that case records were patchy.

Comparisons of data from different levels in the system show that the further away from the disabled person and their direct carers the data gathering is focused, the fewer cases are acknowledged (Brown 1994). For example in a series of studies in the early 1990s in the United Kingdom and Ireland, direct care staff believed that 8% of their adult intellectually disabled clients had been sexually abused, whereas psychiatrists put the figure at 4%. But when asked through intensive interviews approximately 50% of intellectually disabled adults indicated that they had been sexually abused in their lifetime (Brown 1993). What is interesting is not that surveys come up with different figures, but that these discrepancies tell us about which "slices" of the whole picture each service is able to uncover and acknowledge.

This pattern of hidden abuse is also found in relation to older people. A rigorous study of elder abuse carried out in Massachusetts (Pillimer and Finkelhor 1988) suggested that only one in 14 cases were reported to statutory authorities, supporting this "tip of an iceberg" model. A number of factors are thought to influence whether a particular case is likely to come to the attention of service providers. Wolf and Donglin (1999) suggested that elders were more likely to feature in reports to statutory services if they were poor and already previously in contact with statutory service providers. These known welfare clients were already under scrutiny from people with a mandate to pass on concerns. Brown and Stein (1998) in their study of reports of all vulnerable adults also found that 80% of referrals concerned people who were already in touch with social services.

This should lead us to be cautious about interpreting data and inquisitive about cases which are not reported. For example in one United Kingdom study of sexual abuse of intellectually disabled adults (Brown, Turk & Stein 1995) one half of reported cases involved abuse by other disabled service users and approximately 15% abuse by staff. But clearly different contingencies were in operation when it came to detecting abuse by more powerful men who could use threats to enforce the secrecy of what they were doing and plan their abuse to take place where they would not be discovered. Later analysis (Brown & Stein 1997) showed that abuses perpetrated by intellectually disabled men were much more likely to have been witnessed but less serious than those which involved abuse of power and authority. Moreover offences committed by intellectually disabled men were less likely to be dealt with by law enforcement agencies or proceed through the criminal justice system so if a study were to rely on information extracted from records of prosecutions these would not have been noted at all.

Hence although studies often set out to address research questions such as:

- the extent of abuse involving disabled children and adults (i.e. incidence and prevalence);

- whether disabled children and adults are at increased risk when compared to their non-disabled peers;

- whether some groups of disabled children and adults are more at risk than others;

- the characteristics of those cases which are officially reported to responsible agencies.

Many are only able to accurately address the last question and thereby enter their findings into a pool from which it is possible to make some informed and qualified guesses.

3.2. Is abuse increasing?

Caution needs to be exercised when assessing trends. Although the European Disability Forum (EDF) (1999a) marshals evidence to suggest that abuse against people with disabilities is on the increase, it is difficult to determine if abuse of disabled adults and children is actually more frequent or just more likely to be reported or talked about. When care was provided in large segregated settings, scrutiny and regulation were minimal and routes for complaint non-existent. An alternative hypothesis is that abuse is now more visible and more likely to be noted because it occurs in "ordinary" settings, where it is more likely to be judged against normal expectations and assumptions. Also mainstreaming throws up *different* pressures for people with disabilities than those previously experienced in institutional settings: for example in schools it may lead to bullying and in community situations to isolation or harassment. For example a respondent to a recent survey of people with intellectual disabilities (Mencap 1999:15) reported that:

> I live in a council estate [social housing], kids, a group of four or five children, abuse me all the time. One of them has threatened to beat me up when I leave the home to visit my sister. I fancy moving as I can't go on. I cry about it. They make fun of me, they throw stones, they smash up my windows. Last year our gate was broken, and somebody smashed up all the glass windows in our greenhouse. The police won't do anything about it.

Changing expectations also make it difficult to compare studies across time. For example in the United Kingdom physical punishment in schools was not made illegal in state schools until 1986 and was still legal for another ten years in independent (private) schools. These legitimated assaults would not previously have been reported as abuse, nor was sexual abuse registered as a distinct form of abuse until relatively recently (Stevenson 1996).

On the other hand, there is growing concern about verbal abuse in public places and the abuses linked to right wing ideologies (European Disability Forum (EDF) 1999a:9). This rising tide of violence is noted in communities across member states and has been exacerbated by recent upheavals involving the movement of refugees as a result of war, migration and economic policies, which have created greater inequalities within and between countries.

The evidence does however indicate a rise in reporting. Figures from France show increased reporting as a result of more proactive policies and in Alabama (USA) reports under their vulnerable adult statute rose more than tenfold in a ten-year period (from 477 cases in 1978 to 5,220 in 1989; Daniels, Baumhover & Clark-Daniels 1989). The trend in reporting of all child abuse (as opposed to abuse of disabled children specifically) is upwards across member states. Increased reporting reflects increased awareness and competence rather than increasing abuse and it is likely that reports will continue to rise as responsible agencies raise public awareness and make routes for referral clearer.

Sound research in this field needs to be transparent about its scope and limitations and describe for the research community the exact context and circumstances in which data was gathered including:

- How abuse was defined not only on paper but in professional discourse, institutional cultures and through training;

- What was known about this sample or agency and its networks which influenced which victims, perpetrators and types of abuse were likely to be registered;

- The contingencies which might have influenced readiness to report, for example if benefits might be removed from a family which had been abusive one might expect few people to volunteer reports. If, on the other hand, additional respite care were offered to families under pressure they might define situations as potentially abusive in order to be eligible for this service;

- Any problems experienced in relation to data gathering – for example how interviews with persons with communication difficulties were conducted, what level of staff turnover existed in an organisation which is the subject of a retro-spective survey;

• How an ethical dimension was incorporated into the research design so that individuals were not invited to disclose experience of abuse or abusing without being offered support and/or appropriate intervention and nor were they invited to risk incriminating themselves or others in ignorance of any limits to confidentiality: this is particularly important when working with perpetrators who are themselves vulnerable and/or have learning disabilities or mental health problems (see Hall & Osborn 1994: Brown & Thompson 1997a).

These pointers are not intended to cast doubt on existing research in this field but to provide cues for reading it intelligently. They set out a framework for robustness in a field which does not lend itself to more orthodox methodologies. Traditional approaches typically fail to address the complexity of case identification and reporting (see for example Stanko 2000), and tend to downplay the significance of user involvement at all stages of the research process, whether it be defining research priorities or questions, refining data gathering techniques or providing an ethical overview of the conduct of research (Rioux & Bach 1994).

3.3. Cautious findings on abuse of disabled children

These caveats need to be borne in mind when research findings on abuse of disabled children are reviewed. Under-reporting should be assumed in all types of study including thoco which have control groups to estimate differential rates of abuse for disabled girls and boys.

There is evidence to support the view that disabled children are at increased risk. Glaser and Bentovim (1979) pioneers in this field identified higher risks of abuse for disabled and chronically ill children who were patients for other reasons and not referred specifically as result of concerns about abuse. An important American study by Crosse, Kaye and Ratnofsky (1993) collected data on all substantiated cases of child abuse from 35 child protection services across the USA over a six-week period. This data demonstrated an increased risk to disabled children (1.7 times the risk of all children). But even this figure relied on child protection workers to reliably note and describe various disabilities and is thought to have missed children cared for in residential settings. A study in Utrecht revealed that children with a physical disability or chronic illness were also five times as likely to be subjected to bullying at school.

But increased risk does not always filter through as increased reporting. In a study by Kvam (2000) sexual abuse of children in Norway was monitored through the paediatric units to which they are referred for medical examination. Using recent American research as a guide, the researchers expected to see a higher rate of referrals for disabled children but found instead a much lower rate. Overall disabled children form 11% of the relevant population and, if increased risk were reflected would have accounted for about a third of reports but only 6.4% of the total sample of reported cases concerned children with disabilities. The discrepancy was particularly evident for the 4% of the total population of children with severe disabilities who accounted for only 1.7% of referrals. The author suggests that as a group disabled children may be less likely to disclose or to have their disclosures listened to and also that abuse against them is minimised and not taken seriously.

Research in Spain has not generally focused specifically on disabled children but they have been identified within several broader studies (Alonso, Bermejo, Zurito & Simón 1994). One large scale investigation of parenting revealed that almost half of the parents acknowledged at least the occasional use of corporal punishment and that disabled children were not exempt. 6.7% of the children ill-treated by these parents had delayed development or intellectual disabilities and 5.4% behavioural problems (Ortega, González & Cabanillas 1997). A study which did focus on disabled children and young people in Castile identified 51 mistreated children and young people in a sample of 445. The categories of abuse used in this study were slightly broader than the typology we set out in this report. Physical and emotional abandonment were identified as the most frequent types of ill treatment/abuse, followed by emotional and physical abuse, exploitation for work (ie child labour) and sexual abuse.

In line with other studies this study showed that abused children and young people are likely to be subjected to a range of abuse not only one "type". Disabled children were less likely than their peers to be physically abused but correspondingly more likely to be ignored, neglected or abandoned. Nor did the risk diminish as the children got older. Caution must be exercised in seeming to locate the cause of the abusive behaviour with the victims but it was noted that communication difficulties and challenging behaviour were significant factors. Abusing parents were likely to come from lower socio-economic groups, not to have collaborative relationships with different professionals, to have had insufficient knowledge of their child's disability and unrealistic expectations about their future development. Alcohol misuse and marital violence also played a part. A correlation was also noted between the level of material deprivation suffered by the family and the seriousness of the abuse.

Other important information has been gleaned from studies which address issues for both adults and children. Sobsey (1994) hypothesised, as a result of a Canadian survey, that the increased rate of sexual abuse to disabled children and adults derived from the increased statistical risk of encountering an abuser through their contact with multiple service providers in the context of personal care. Major inquiries into service breakdowns and court cases also yield important data although these may not be routinely collated and analysed from the perspective of disabled children.

3.4. Cautious findings on abuse of disabled adults

There is conflicting evidence as to whether disabled adults are at greater risk of violence and assault than other members of the general population. Analysis of the 1996 British Crime Survey (which includes unreported crime but excludes people living in residential care) suggested that once other factors such as nature of housing, age and time spent out of the home were controlled for, people with disabilities were at no extra risk. However data from Australia suggested that people with intellectual disabilities may be at increased risk of both personal (2x) and property (1.5x) crimes (Australian Bureau of Statistics 1986; Wilson & Brewer 1992). Many studies focus on specific types of abuse, client groups or settings.

3.4.1. Sexual abuse

Following in the wake of much greater awareness of the sexual abuse of children both within and beyond their families and an increasing understanding of sexual offending as a compulsive behaviour usually, but not exclusively, perpetrated by men, sexual abuse has been highlighted in relation to people with learning disabilities (Turk & Brown 1993; Brown, Stein & Turk 1995; Zijdel 1999), in relation to deaf women and children (Merkin & Smith 1995) and in relation to people using mental health services especially counsellors and therapists (Schoener *et al.* 1989; Penfold 1998). Penfold specifically likens sexual involvement between powerful health professionals and their clients to incestuous sexual relationships.

Sexual abuse has a distinct aetiology and gendered pattern. Abusers tend to repeat their offences and actively seek out victims. This raises very particular issues in terms of prevention in line with current concern in relation to paedophilia and child sexual abuse and exploitation. Abuse is usually carried out by men within the person's network and not by strangers; perpetrators are predominantly men but a significant minority of victims are also men. No single group emerge as more likely victims other than those who live or spend their time alongside abusers, but a consistent power dynamic emerges whether centred on authority, gender, physical or intellectual ability (Thompson 1997).

Findings on sexual violence are available from a number of studies in member states as well as from North American and Canadian surveys. Van Berlo (1995) from the Netherlands found that of a total population of approximately 100,000 people with intellectual disabilities 1,100 people had been victims of sexual abuse in the previous two years and a further 1,200 of suspected sexual abuse. Of the victims 4/5 were women while the perpetrators were predominantly men. The findings of a United Kingdom study (Turk & Brown 1993; Brown, Stein & Turk 1995) and this study from the Netherlands are broadly consistent. The United Kingdom study noted a higher proportion of male victims.

As to the perpetrators, one third in Van Berlo's study were other service users as were one half of those in the United Kingdom study and they were seen to have offended against more male victims proportionately (see also van den Bergh, Hoekema & van der Ploeg 1997). Other offenders included parents, spouses, relatives, neighbours, service personnel, transport and domestic workers, professionals, church workers and educators (see van den Bergh, Hoekema & van der Ploeg 1997). Similar patterns of abusing, often featuring active targeting and grooming of potential victims, were reported even where the offenders were learning disabled themselves (see Thompson & Brown 1998; Churchill, Brown, Horrocks & Craft 1997), although there was evidence that learning disabled men were less sophisticated/successful and more likely to be witnessed in their offending behaviour (Brown & Stein 1997). Studies which have focused on the disclosures of people with intellectual disabilities themselves as opposed to reports to service agencies report a higher proportion of offences committed by family members than the services are aware of (McCarthy & Thompson 1997). They also found higher levels of abuse supporting the "tip of the iceberg" hypothesis and illustrating how reports get filtered out and/or ignored within service agencies. Cases which do come to court represent the pinnacle of this iceberg, for example in Slovenia 17 such cases were registered by the police in 1999 while six persons where sentenced by court (note of the Slovenian delegation; see also van den Bergh, Douma & Hoekema 1999 for information about the interface between the police and victims/perpetrators with intellectual disabilities).

While abuse of people with learning disabilities raises particular legal and ethical issues these concerns are matched by evidence that other disabled groups are also at heightened risk of sexual abuse. Several sources suggest that deaf children and adults are particularly at risk and that deaf women are at greater risk of domestic violence than other women (Merkin & Smith 1995). This should filter through onto the curriculum for deaf pupils and also onto the professional curricula of social workers who need both deaf- awareness and abuse-awareness training and access to skilled interpreters who can combine signing competency with awareness of the effects of abuse and the demands of the court system. Other child and adult protection specialists have developed strategies for enabling children who use alternative forms of communication to make statements and testify against their abusers (Marchant & Page 1992).

Sexual involvement of adults in therapy – a one-to-one intense relationship often carried out in private and without supervision – has been harder to conceptualise and has sometimes been rationalised as sex between consenting adults or blamed on "seductive" victims. As Penfold (1998:169) comments, this ignores *"the vast power differential between health professional and patient, the fiduciary relationship, and the parent-like role of the professional"*. This power imbalance may also be enshrined in law with the professional having legal powers to detain or restrain. This obviously makes for a very difficult research environment and task, given that victims may feel, and actually are, at risk of being discredited or blamed for their predicament and may be unwilling to come forward for fear of being shamed. Research has actually been more forthcoming when health professionals themselves have been anonymously surveyed. Various studies cited by Penfold (1998:10) suggest that 3-4% male professionals report their own involvement in exploitative sexual relationships and 0.5-1% of female professionals. A British study of psychologists (Garrett 1998) arrived at a similar figure.

3.4.2. Physical abuse

Although sexual abuse has been in the limelight, studies involving all vulnerable adult client groups suggest that physical abuse is more common and more likely to grow out of the daily stresses of care and out of unskilled attempts to control and manage the environment. The gender imbalance seen in sexual abusing is not evident. Physical abuse also is more likely to be triggered by naïve approaches to serious challenging behaviours and to an adherence to popular child-rearing beliefs about the efficacy of physical punishment. Because the acts and situations under this heading are so broad few incidence studies have been attempted – a low level of physical abuse is almost accepted as endemic in institutions, residential homes and day centres. Research has focused more on trying to identify patterns and causes and has drawn on qualitative as well as quantitative methodologies.

Cambridge (1999) described an abusive service providing intensive care to two people with challenging behaviours and analysed the causes of the abuse at four levels: in terms of the individuals' complex needs, the support and procedures required by direct care staff, the professional advice and input required, and the management arrangements for regulation and supervision. In the absence of good practice at all these levels the regime which was allowed to emerge around these two service users was characterised by controlling and punitive approaches: new inexperienced staff were inducted into a regime in which they were told they would have no problems after "the first hit". Outsiders were excluded on the basis that this preserved privacy and "homeliness" but it also allowed this situation to continue without independent scrutiny.

Findings on physical abuse may be masked by alternative discourses and terminology. For example, it is acknowledged that difficult or violent behaviour may be part of the presenting problem which leads someone to use services or require institutional care. In services for people with intellectual disabilities a non-blaming stance has been successful in de-stigmatising such behaviour and mobilising consistent responses

77

from staff groups. Nevertheless, behaviour which is described as "challenging behaviour" may include frequent assaults on other service users, as well as on staff and/or self harming. Victims of such assaults may not receive support and protection because the service is keen to avoid a punitive stance towards those responsible. Conversely, several studies suggest that people with challenging behaviours or autism are most at risk of physical abuse (Foubert 1998) because restraining measures and controlling strategies tip over into punitive practice and provide a spurious rationale for retaliation.

3.4.3. Research across different types of abuse

Brown and Stein (1998) analysed reports under the generic adult protection policies of two large local authorities in South-east England, subsequently replicated in 10 further authorities (Brown and Stein 2000). They documented a reporting rate of 20-25 cases per 100,000 general population over the age of 18, per annum, of which about one third of referrals concern people with intellectual disabilities, and a further one third of cases cover people with physical, sensory and mental health problems and people who are ill (the remaining one third of cases referred to older people). Different profiles of abuse were registered for these client groups with more sexual abuse being reported for intellectually disabled people and more financial abuse noted amongst older clients. But to some extent these differences reflect practice and awareness as well as real differences in risk. These reports did not rely on assertive outreach but in the vast majority of cases referred to clients who were already known to service agencies.

Of equal importance is the finding that in one fifth of cases multiple abuses were noted, demonstrating the need to look carefully at all manifestations of cruelty and disrespect within a relationship or setting rather than be blinkered by labels and categories (see also Ministère de l'emploi et de la solidarité 1998). Other studies have concentrated on different settings and contexts. A recent United Kingdom study on bullying (harassment) in people's neighbourhoods and communities reported widespread verbal abuse overlapping with physical abuse in public places (Mencap 1999).

3.5. Individual and structural causes of abuse

An initial reading of some of these studies tends to favour explanations which focus on the impact of individual impairment, the behaviour of individual offenders or cruelty within particular families. But social factors can be seen to exacerbate these tendencies especially where abuse takes place within institutions and other service settings. Zijdel (1999:20-23), in her contribution to a conference marking the 1999 European Day of Disabled People, identified factors at all levels including lack of education, isolation, deprivation of information, economic dependence, low self-esteem and political and legislative unawareness. To this we would also add lack of knowledge on the part of staff especially those working with people who have complex needs such as autism or challenging behaviour (Cachemaille 2000:10).

Valuable data also emerge from one-off inquiries and court cases which tend to provide a more in-depth account of the dynamics and culture of those establishments in which standards have declined. A recent review of a serious case in the United Kingdom (Buckinghamshire County Council 1998) revealed a catalogue of abuses and cruelty by the proprietor/ director of the establishment exacerbated by the fact that his staff had little knowledge or expertise to equip them to work with clients who had a range of challenging behaviours. Instead of properly accountable practice and behavioural programmes the regime relied on bullying and punishment such as:

- leaving people outside in the cold;
- making someone who had difficulty with feeding eat her meals outside;
- sending people to their rooms;
- rationing their toiletries and toilet paper;
- mismanaging their money;
- occasionally hitting them.

79

Although in this case it seemed at first that the problem resided with this individual, a closer analysis indicated that many common features of institutional living had played a part, if not in motivating his behaviour, then at least in allowing it to continue unchallenged. Moreover it could be seen that he had operated to maximise his own power by employing his wife as deputy and other relatives or unqualified staff, and by cynically joining charitable and political networks in order to close down avenues for complaints which might otherwise have been routed through influential local public figures.

An inquiry of even greater scope recently took place in North Wales (Waterhouse Inquiry 2000) which uncovered widespread and systematic abuse in children's homes across several counties and addressed failures in management and in the regulatory framework which allowed some of the most vulnerable young people in the care system to go unheard. These young people, often characterised as delinquent rather than vulnerable, were brought back to abusive regimes when they ran away, discredited when they gave accounts of their abuse and not afforded any independent advocacy or protection from the law. Their abuse took place against a backdrop of ignorance about the serial nature of paedophilia and about the strategies paedophiles use to access potential victims and gradually groom them into keeping silent about abuse while systematically closing off avenues for them to disclose. Lessons can also be learned from the "pindown" inquiry which investigated routine breaches of human rights and abuse of "grounding" and restraint practices in children's homes and which laid the way for proper guidance in this area (Staffordshire County Council 1991).

Of most significance in these studies are attempts to locate causes. Goffman's (1961) original treatise on institutionalisation still provides a useful analysis, using concepts of depersonalisation and routine. More recent studies have focused on the split between unqualified and low-paid workers who do the bulk of the physical work in such settings (see for example Wardhaugh and Wilding 1993) and their managers or professional advisors who, despite their knowledge base and expertise, spend least time with the most difficult client groups. The European Committee for the Prevention of Torture and Inhuman or Degrading Treatment or Punishment (CPT) (1998) notes that ill-treatment in psychiatric hospitals tends to be by orderlies rather than medical staff. Recent research in the United Kingdom identified private care homes as the most frequent flouter of minimum wage legislation (Hetherington 2000), so that appeals to high-sounding values and mission statements may ring hollow with workers who are themselves being exploited.

Lee-Treweek (1994) points to the hierarchical relations between qualified staff and orderlies and documents the sub-culture which emerges in these conditions. Low-paid staff do the feeding, toileting and dressing tasks often unsupported by those more skilled professional staff who remain at "arms length" and are able to hide behind ideals and rhetoric which they never have to put into practice. Those with most knowledge often interact with people with disabilities for relatively short periods of time. Moreover the person directly responsible for any abuse may be the scapegoat in the whole system where services are left understaffed and/or staff are not given sufficient training, adequate resources or an adequate knowledge base from which to care for clients with complex needs and demanding behaviour.

The discourse of abuse tends to point towards explanations at the level of individual wrongdoing but clearly there are structural issues which cannot, and should not, be ignored in these situations which include

• resource constraints and staffing levels;
• staff who are poorly selected, qualified, trained, supported and paid;
• inadequate inspection and regulation.

Moreover, at a societal level, we have already seen that discriminatory attitudes towards people with disabilities help to create a climate in which abuse against people with disabilities is allowed to continue while at the same time broader social inequalities also conspire to tip the balance against equal and respectful treatment. Gender is one such form of oppression and a specialist report for the Council of Europe examining causes of violence against women explores over-laying factors of power and control vested in people and places:

> "[that is] why some locations and relationships seem particularly conducive to sexual violence: male family members and women's/girls' homes; authority relations and residential settings and state institutions (of particular concern here are orphanages, children's homes, mental hospitals, prisons, and residential homes for disabled and/or elderly women). What is common to these is a combination of gender and other power/authority relations, father/husband, professional, state functionary."
>
> (Group of Specialists for combating violence against women 1997: 15)

The note from France also identifies causes at a range of levels including psychodynamic issues, insufficient commitment, educational strategies, the dynamic of finding scape-goats, social relationships between staff, lack of respect for residents' rights, the extent to which the institution is integrated into the community, and resistance to change. Penfold (1998:85) cites various explanations of boundary violation in professional relationships including indulgence of professional privilege, role reversal where the client takes over responsibility for the practitioner's feelings, secrecy often masquerading as confidentiality and a double bind, for example where attempts to expose or resolve the situation incur penalties or abandonment.

Several researchers have found it useful to conceptualise the abuse as a series of concentric circles representing the influence of different layers of oppression, each of which have a bearing on the individual interaction which is identified as overtly abusive (see for example Wardhaugh & Wilding 1993; Cambridge 1999). Hence a general societal devaluing of people with disabilities may lead to low levels of resources being assigned to their care, which may in turn translate to a few low-paid staff being on duty who do not know how to deal appropriately with a challenging client. The abusive incident becomes an almost inevitable link in a chain reaction of disadvantage.

3.6. Generating comparable data across member states

Because research is in its infancy, routine evaluation and comparison of responses, treatment and service options have not been carried out across member states. One goal of this report is to stimulate the collection and analysis of data and provide the raw material for shared systematic review and research across member states. In order to do that, data must be routinely generated and collated.

Data are often unnecessarily hidden in official statistics and returns, for example where figures are compiled about general populations, disabled children and adults may not be identified. Figures collected by generic agencies such as child protection services often do not identify disabled children or note the nature of their disability. In a United Kingdom study of how disabled children fare within generic child protection services (Cooke 1999) only 14% of social services departments could give a figure relating to disabled children who had been abused in the previous year: one third of authorities had separate policies highlighting the needs of disabled children, one half did note when children had a disability although a smaller number specified which type of disability and only a third routinely recorded the presence of a disabled sibling in families about which concerns had been raised. A recent document from the United Kingdom Department of Health (1999b) has urged authorities to adopt more standardised methods of planning and recording in relation to disabled children. Disabled children need to be identified clearly in national statistics about all abused children, including those who are removed from family settings as a result of significant risk of harm who are impaired as a result of this initial mistreatment. Disabled adults are similarly hidden as a sub-group within statistics about crime and personal violence and in returns from refuges and counselling services.

Because this information is not readily available, knowledge about abuse of disabled children and adults lags behind the rest of the field and research is, as a consequence, unduly cumbersome and expensive. Member countries may want to establish whether it is possible to pick out instances involving disabled children and adults from routine statistics as detailed in the checklist at the end of this section.

Recent United Kingdom Government guidance (Department of Health 2000) requires social services departments to set up systems which allow them to collate the following information about referrals concerning vulnerable adults (including elders):

- Number and source of referrals across a given catchment area/population (to produce a comparable rate of reporting);
- Information about the abused person such as age, gender and client group (to assist in monitoring disability, gender and ethnicity);
- Whether the person was already known to helping agencies (to assist in identifying outreach / new referrals);
- Type(s) of abuse which triggered the referral;
- Location and setting of the abuse;
- Information about the perpetrator including gender, relationship, position;
- Number of investigations and case conference;
- Outcomes of investigation;
- User views of whether protective services helped them and whether interventions were acceptable.

Promoting collaboration in research will assist in the development of shared conventions in categorisation and documentation of abuse across all countries and settings, enabling outcomes to be compared and learning to be shared (see, for example, UNAPEI 2000). This collaboration need not be confined to empirical research but also to service development and programme evaluation.

One such collaboration has been in operation between two sex eduationalists specialising in sex education for disabled persons in French-speaking Switzerland, in co-operation with the University of Namur in Belgium (Psychology Department of the Faculty of Medicine). The programme is called *Des femmes et des hommes* (Of women and men) and is aimed at intellectually disabled adults and young people (Delville, Mercier & Merlin 2000). Another programme for educators and care staff has been drawn up by the same educationalists (Agthe Diserens & Vatre 2000a). The programme, entitled *Du coeur au corps, ou Formons-nous ... puis formons-les* (From the heart to the body, or let's train ourselves ... then train them) was awarded the Swiss Prize for Remedial Education in 2001.

This kind of partnership is seen as an important way forward in sharing knowledge about solutions as well as about the nature and extent of the problem.

3.7. Summary and checklist

Learning from research: While it is impossible to establish exact figures for **incidence** (number of reports in a given time span) or **prevalence** (percentage of people with disabilities abused at some time during their lifetime) or for raised levels of risk, it is possible to say that people with disabilities are exposed to *at least the same and probably more risk of abuse* as other people and that they require *at least the same level of protection* and access to redress.

1. In your country has rigorous research been carried out to identify the extent and nature of abuse against all major client groups covered within this report:

- children with physical impairments;
- children with sensory impairments and/or alternative communication systems;
- children with mental health problems;
- children and adults with autism;
- people with intellectual disabilities (both severe/profound and mild/moderate);

85

- people with mental health problems including those with severe and enduring mental health problems;

- young people with mental health problems including those who have found their way into the welfare system because they have committed offences;

- adults with physical and mobility problems including those living independently and managing their own care;

- adults with sensory impairments and alternative communication strategies.

2.   It is hypothesised that the following factors contribute to increased risk:

- public hostility or indifference to people who are visibly different;

- institutional cultures, regimes and structures in which direct care staff have low skills, status and pay; where there is resistance to change and a closed community; unequal pay, conditions and training opportunities for qualified and unqualified staff;

- repeated exposure to multiple carers for those in receipt of personal assistance and intimate care;

- ignorance and poor training of staff who work with people who have complex needs and/or challenging behaviours;

- lack of regulation or strong accountability to an independent agency/ department.

Are **services routinely inspected or evaluated** to see if these factors are a feature of life in residential care or day centres for citizens of your country/region?

3.   Impairment does not in itself make people vulnerable although communication or credibility difficulties, sensory and cognitive impairments, may signal to potential abusers the idea that people with disabilities are "safe" people to victimise: failure to apply the criminal justice system on behalf of people with disabilities confirms this assessment. Are details about **criminal proceedings** involving people with disabilities

and vulnerable children or adults routinely collated and audited in order to learn how best to facilitate courtroom practice and to maximise access to justice?

4. **Sexual abusing** is usually a serial type of offending and difficult to change or stop without clear intervention and careful supervision: risk management of sexual offenders and preventing them from coming into contact with disabled children and adults is an important service responsibility. Sexual abuse (unlike other forms of abuse) has a gendered pattern with men forming the majority of perpetrators but both women and men being victimised by them. "Grooming" is a process whereby a person is targeted and made the focus of the perpetrator's attentions and gradually drawn into the abusive relationship.

Are there any current research projects in your country/region which explore sexual offending and sexually exploitative behaviour (with a view to preventing it) in the following contexts:

• special education including boarding schools for disabled children and young people;

• services for people with learning disabilities;

• services for people with mental health problems;

• professional or therapeutic relationships;

• pastoral care and church work;

• voluntary work and leisure/ holiday clubs;

• community settings and ordinary employment?

5. Financial abuse might also involve deliberate targeting and/or a gradual testing of limits.

• Has research been funded to explore safeguards and advocacy in relation to financial matters for different client groups who are the subject of this report?

6. **Institutional models** of care and service structures weaken family and community networks thereby **undermining important sources of support and protection** for disabled children and adults.

- Are independent inquiries held and published into services or settings which fail or in which abuse is alleged or uncovered?

- Is there a programme of de-institutionalisation in progress in your country and if so is this being supported/evaluated by a partnership of academic and service provider organisations?

7. Is **user involvement** usually incorporated into funding criteria and research proposals at all stages of the research process, including:

- debating and deciding upon the research agenda;

- defining research priorities;

- prioritising research questions;

- refining data-gathering techniques;

- providing an ethical overview of the conduct of research;

- disseminating and implementing findings?

8. Disabled children and adults are often invisible in routine data-gathering to inform social policy. In your country are **disabled persons systematically identified** in:

- child protection reports, care orders and "place of safety orders";

- admissions to accident and emergency units where non-accidental injury is identified;

- returns about victims of crime, particularly crimes against the person and sexual crime;

- use of mainstream services designed to assist people in dealing with issues of abuse, eg referrals to rape crisis services, incest survivors groups, help lines;

- where residential services are inspected and regulated, in statistics relating to complaints and home closures involving people with disabilities?

9. How is **research funding** organised to facilitate studies of abuse and abusing in your country?

- Is there a routine stream of funding for research into disabled people's issues and services which includes abuse and protection issues?

- Is research funded by agencies or interest groups who might downplay or have conflicts of interest in research in this arena, for example, by the church or by proprietors of services or particular professional groups?

- Do people with disabilities get their fair share of mainstream research funding in relation to their health care issues, experiences of the criminal justice system, community safety, access to justice and to employment?

- Are users and their organisations involved in research funding decisions?

- Are safeguards around consent, free choice to be involved or not, and civil rights, routinely built into all research proposals involving disabled persons as subjects of that research?

- Are protection and abuse issues built into funding criteria for key areas of work, for example service evaluation, assessment, challenging behaviour?

4. THE ROLE OF LAW IN PROTECTING PEOPLE WITH DISABILITIES

4.1. The role of law

This document is not primarily concerned with legislative change but the legal framework and enforcement process plays an important part in the protection of people with disabilities by enshrining rights and safeguards in legislation and by providing important avenues through which people with disabilities can seek redress. Specific offences set clear boundaries around what is acceptable and may provide additional safeguards for the most vulnerable people. The law also provides the basis for the involvement of the state by defining (and limiting) the powers and the duties of public bodies to intervene in the lives of individual citizens.

The European Convention on Human Rights provides an important benchmark in this respect and any changes necessary to strengthen the position of vulnerable children and adults in the laws of member states should be set firmly within this framework. Two important principles flow from this commitment to human rights:

- formal *equality* of disabled children and adults and entitlement to *equivalent* treatment in law and health care with whatever assistance they need to pursue and uphold this (Article 6);

- *proportionality* and independent *scrutiny* of any controlling, protective or limiting approaches, for example where detention or restraint is thought to be in the best interests of a disabled person and/or necessary to secure their immediate safety or the protection of others, or where people with disabilities might be considered to be at risk of exploitation and unable to consent to certain transactions.

Disabled Peoples' International (DPI) has a Human Rights Task Force currently active in five member states consisting of volunteer co-ordinators who are collecting data nationally about breaches of this legislation (Gooding 1998).

These protections work at different levels, in relation to:

- the *definition* of abuse against people with disabilities through the use of generic criminal codes and where laws specify circumstances or acts which are illegal in relation to people with disabilities, for example sexual or financial exploitation;

- the part that law plays in *prevention* of abuse either directly or by setting up safeguards in services which make abuse of people with disabilities less likely. This law includes, for example, legislation about the standards and regulation of professionals and care settings; legal processes to evaluate the use of unwarranted force or detention and a framework to limit or mandate the appropriate sharing of information;

- access to the criminal or civil law to provide *redress* and/or compensation to people with disabilities who have been victims of violence and to punish wrongdoers which, in itself, sends important signals that the community values people with disabilities and will act to protect them. Access to justice is an important element of civil liberties and redress should be available through ordinary routes with additional assistance where this is necessary such as in helping individuals to give evidence in court and to participate in the legal process without being intimidated (see Home Office 1998; European Disability Forum 1999a:14-15).

The legal systems of member states vary considerably, some drawing on an inquisitorial, and others an adversarial tradition. Given that the report cannot provide a detailed overview what follows is a series of pointers and models to assist member states in reviewing their own legislation in order to identify gaps and priorities. It is also important to note that judges, police officers, probation officers and other professionals working within the criminal justice system will have considerable training needs if they are to begin to offer a more inclusive and less discriminatory approach to people with disabilities whether as victims, witnesses or offenders or as applicants under civil law to have their rights upheld (see Département de la prévoyance sociale et des assurances 1996 and 1998 for conference reports on these issues).

4.2. Definitions of abusive acts

The rights of people with disabilities are codified in a number of important international documents and declarations but these are enshrined differentially in national laws and in practice. It should be taken as read that people with disabilities are included, alongside all citizens, in the general criminal code which outlaws personal and sexual violence, theft and other threatening behaviours. In some countries women and minority ethnic groups may be protected by additional specific legislation. Attitudes to domestic violence vary across member states (see Swedish Social Services Act 1998, section 8a which promises support to women who are victims of domestic violence; Swedish Social Services Department 1998). Where violence against people with disabilities is specifically mentioned there may be a specific responsibility for reporting concerns to the relevant authorities (see Swedish Social Services Act 1998, section 71a). Mandatory reporting has been a central plank of American Vulnerable Adults' Statutes and of mainstream child protection systems.

Several countries have incorporated the European Convention on Human Rights into their legislative frameworks and concerns which have flowed from this include action on children's rights and on conditions in psychiatric hospitals. In Hungary an inquiry was set up in 1997 to look into inhuman conditions in institutions in that country and measures were promised to improve the situation. The Spanish Constitution has adopted the anti-discrimination principle and devised a quality assurance programme in relation to social services to support it.

4.2.1. Informed consent

Consent and capacity are important concepts when defining abuse as it affects individual adults with disabilities (Law Commission 1995: Murphy & Clare 1995). While the laws of member states make a blanket assumption that children are not able to enter into sexual or financial transactions, for example by naming an "age of consent" for sexual acts or making valid contracts, disabled adults vary in their capacity to enter into, and protect themselves within, such agreements. It is important that legislation designed to protect people with disabilities does not cut across a commitment to uphold their civil liberties in sexual and economic relationships. The United Kingdom Law Commission suggested the following test to be used.

> "A person should be regarded as unable to make a decision by reason of disability if it is such that, at the time when the decision needs to be made, he or she is either unable to understand or retain, or make a decision based on, relevant information including information about reasonably foreseeable consequences of deciding one way or the other, or failing to make the decision" (clause 2(2) of the Draft Bill on Mental Incapacity, Law Commission 1995).

However, sometimes the duty to protect is abdicated on the false assumption that non-intervention equates to autonomy whereas sometimes action is needed in order to safeguard an individual's autonomy. Moody (1988) proposed a shift from "informed" to "negotiated" consent as the guiding principle in long term care services for older people and this might be extended to some of the situations faced by people with disabilities. He (1988:64) argued that:

> *"autonomy and paternalism, commonly understood as opposites, need not, in fact, be opposed at all. In the environment of long-term care ... paternalistic interventions are called for that serve to enhance autonomy; namely the capacity of patients [sic] to decide and to act in keeping with their own values. Thinking about paternalistic intervention in this way, it becomes clear that the informed consent standard is an impoverished guideline for professionals to use in thinking about the moral dilemmas ...*

[and] needs to be replaced by a more subtle and complex set of standards or what could be called negotiated consent".

The notion of valid and informed consent hinges on the capacity to

- indicate consent in a given situation;
- to be adequately informed and understand enough about the consequences of the decision (for example the European Committee for the Prevention of Torture and Inhuman or Degrading Treatment or Punishment (CPT) argues that it is not sufficient to tell a patient that they are to have a "sleeping treatment" to ascertain their valid consent to ECT);
- and remain free from undue pressure or coercion from others when making the decision, especially when those urging compliance are also those who provide every day care and/or control.

Ability to consent will therefore be affected by the commitment and expertise of professionals to provide accessible information. Interpreters are needed for persons who use sign language and to facilitate augmented communication for those with limited speech. Educational interventions such as social skills training and sex education enables people to make better informed choices about their lives while independent advocacy provides a safeguard in the process of decision making which is particularly important where people with disabilities are having to make decisions in service settings or in the presence of authority figures.

The law also takes a view about what may be consented to and may stipulate a degree of harm or violence which lies beyond the possibility of valid consent (see Law Commission 1995:214-44 for a comparison of different legal systems in relation to this issue). The notion of "consent" in this respect is critical because the law otherwise allows the individual to waive the right to prosecution in more minor assaults but this principle may be misapplied to situations in which vulnerable children or adults are too intimidated to be able to make a valid choice to forego the protection of law. Children and young people are specifically deemed not to be able to give consent to certain categories of decision.

For example Council of Europe Parliamentary Assembly Recommendation 1371 (1998) urges member states to declare unequivocally that prostitution of minors (under 15) *"always constitutes rape or sexual abuse and that, even where money has been handed over, there is a presumption of violence since a child cannot be regarded as a consenting party"* (c.i). Persons with severe intellectual disabilities are deemed not to be able to give consent to sexual or financial transactions in the United Kingdom and in other countries. People with mental health problems may move in and out of mental states which allow them to make sound decisions.

4.2.2. Capacity to make decisions

In most countries, for example Estonia, there is an assumption of capacity unless a court has ruled that the person is not able to manage their affairs. This ruling may apply to all areas of the person's life or to more specific decisions. A form of guardianship exists in Italy whereby someone is appointed to administer specific aspects of an individual's affairs until such time as they are able to manage on their own. Mental incapacity legislation exists in several other member states including Belgium which declares an individual of "extended minority" if a person is unable to administer their affairs after the age of 18. This provides a form of guardianship analogous to the United Kingdom's Court of Protection which oversees the administration of a disabled person's property and income. When the person's affairs are being managed by service providers there is a need for independent scrutiny. Following a recent independent inquiry into ongoing abuses at a residential home in Buckinghamshire (United Kingdom) the government stipulated that home owners or manager should not be entrusted with the management of clients' monies as a matter of principle. Following the Flemish community and this recent United Kingdom case it is recommended that administration of property and assets should be independent of whichever agency manages a disabled person's day-to-day care and accommodation.

Certain decisions are deemed too important and irreversible for children or persons without mental capacity to make without extra safeguards in the form of judicial hearing/review. For example "sterilisation of a minor is limited to only those cases in which reproduction would occasion a serious risk and then under judicial review only and with additional safeguards in the form of agreement by the minor's legal representatives and a panel of three doctors under recommendation" (Council of Europe Parliamentary Assembly 1998:g.ii). This principle extends to adults who lack capacity to make such a decision. A United Kingdom court case in which a mother was given permission to have her 28 year-old daughter sterilised was appealed by the Official Solicitor who "acts for those unable to look after their own legal interests" on the grounds that

> The issue is whether a less invasive method of treatment is in her best interests ... The woman's 54 year-old mother, a widow, fears her daughter could become pregnant when she moves into a residential home, either through forming an emotional attachment with another resident, or through somebody taking advantage of her or raping her. She wanted her daughter to have a hysterectomy because this would not only protect her from pregnancy but also stop her periods altogether. But the Official Solicitor argued that a Mirena coil would be a simpler, easier and less invasive operation.
>
> (Guardian Newspaper 28 January 2000)

In some countries "capacity" is dealt with by declaring adults who cannot make decisions unaided to be legal "minors" and regard their issues as analogous to those of children (e.g. Belgium see above). While this provides one model of protection it does so at the risk of infantilising all disabled adults and inadvertently implying that they are childlike in other aspects of their lives. Adult status is an important badge of citizenship for disabled persons as it is for all citizens. An alternative approach for member states to consider is legislation which provides mechanisms which allow the functional capacity of vulnerable adults to be formally assessed and reviewed in relation to specific decisions and protection issues.

A recommendation of the Committee of Ministers of the Council of Europe (1999) urges member states to make legislative provision for people lacking mental capacity that, as far as possible, preserves the autonomy of individuals and ensures "that a measure of protection should not result automatically in a complete removal of legal capacity". This phrasing of help and protection is in contrast to previous models which polarized individuals as either having capacity or not. Many people with disabilities may lack capacity in some but not all arenas of decision-making and may require action to be taken on their behalf only when they are out of their depth. Others have capacity to make their own decisions but they may still require assistance to access support and assistance if they are being victimized.

4.3. Prevention of abuse and additional safeguards

4.3.1. Detention and compulsory treatment

The European Convention on Human Rights sets out strict conditions under which detention may be authorised – *Article 5 (1) e sets out the right of "persons of unsound mind" not to be deprived of their liberty except in accordance with a procedure prescribed by law.*

According to the European Court of Human Rights the detention of a person of unsound mind is lawful only where,

- a true mental disorder is objectively established;

- the disorder warrants detention and;

- the detention continues no longer than the disorder.

The article also asserts that compulsory treatment in the community will be lawful if it is "proportionate" and "necessary for the protection of health". Article 5 (4) concerns the right of a detained person to take legal proceedings to appeal the lawfulness of his detention and the principle that these appeals should be decided "speedily" by the court. Article 3 of Protocol 1 assures that even detained patients retain the right to vote.

Many countries have legal powers in relation to mentally people with disabilities enshrined in law. These, like the United Kingdom 1983 Mental Health Act specify when it is allowable to use force, to detain someone in a mental hospital for their own safety or for the safety of others and to force them to accept medical treatment for their mental illness or impairment. Detention under this act is only permissible where risk to the individual or to others is deemed to be significant. A recent controversial review of mental health legislation in the United Kingdom extended powers of compulsory treatment but also set out a number of specific safeguards which should be accorded to people who are formally detained; these include

> the right to receive the approved care and treatment and ongoing care for a determined period ... [and] at the earliest opportunity, the right to advocacy, the right to information about and assistance with drawing up an advance agreement and, for those detained in hospital, the right to safe containment consistent with respect for human dignity.
>
> (Department of Health 1999: para 6)

A Tribunal provides independent scrutiny of these decisions and the treatment decisions that flow from them. France has similar legislation. Often people are persuaded to enter asylums voluntarily in which case no formal assessment or hearing may be held. Formality is a double-edged sword. On the one hand, it is cumbersome and can be stigmatising, on the other, it provides an opportunity for assumptions and decisions to be tested and challenged. Additional safeguards are also provided when compulsory treatment is being proposed although there is a great deal of contention around compulsory treatments especially in community settings (United Kingdom) and in relation to Electro Convulsive Therapy (ECT). User representatives at the European Day of Disabled Persons (1999) on Preventing Violence against people with disabilities urged consultation with user groups to build more safeguards into the system and advance directives are under consideration in some states whereby individuals set out, while they are well, how they wish to be treated in crisis situations.

4.3.2. Regulation of workers and settings

Staff with criminal offences and/or unsuitable work records are routinely screened in some states before they are allowed to take up employment which gives them access to children and a position of authority in relation to them. Such mechanisms are in place across member states in relation to children but fewer countries have such a system in operation for those working with adults who might also be at risk of abuse. Norway for example operates a "good conduct" certificate scheme (which certifies that a person has not committed certain crimes) for workers in children's services but not for adults. France has recently adopted a law making it unlawful for anyone convicted of any crime involving bodily harm to work with children or vulnerable adults. Governments should take an overview of such provisions and not allow them to grow in a piecemeal or uncoordinated fashion. Governments also have a role to play in setting up a proper statutory framework for the regulation of professions, including for the accreditation of individuals and the quality assurance of qualifying training, which should include curricula on abuse.

Some member states have laws which regulate settings in which vulnerable people are accommodated and which allow for independent visits and enforcement of adequate standards. Such legislation may, in addition to the powers set out, provide safeguards and/ or avenues for independent review of decisions taken under legislation. The United Kingdom Registered Homes Act 1983 requires all residential accommodation to meet certain standards or face action which can include closure in extreme circumstances. Proprietors and managers of such homes are required to be "fit" persons and their credentials are checked when they initially register their premises. It is unclear in law what constitutes "fitness": prior to opening the home their criminal and professional records are checked and they are subject to an interview but they are not required to hold any specific professional qualification.

After opening their home they may be deemed unfit if they do not manage staff properly or behave appropriately to clients. Currently national standards are being redrawn in a major overhaul of this Act aimed to equalise treatment across the country where previously there was local variation. Day centres are currently outside the regulatory framework although they also may fall into institutional practices and/or be run in substandard premises. Other countries have similar legislation to ensure independent visits to otherwise isolated establishments. France and Belgium have similar independent inspection/regulatory systems.

4.3.3. Regulation of control and restraint

Control and restraint is an issue in many services and may or may not be specifically legislated for (see Harris 1996). Issues came to light in the United Kingdom as a result of a major inquiry into practice in mainstream children's homes which became known as "pindown" and which included solitary confinement in that children were kept alone in their night clothes as punishment for misdemeanours (Staffordshire County Council 1991). A line is not always clearly drawn between control and restraint procedures as a legitimate way of "containing" difficult behaviour to make a person(s) safe in a crisis situation or a covert way of punishing difficult individuals. The manager of this service declared that the regime was based on the principle of "establishing control" but the unequivocal judgment of the Inquiry Team was that this *"stemmed initially from an ill-digested understanding of behavioural psychology" and that "the regime had no theoretical framework and no safeguards"* (Staffordshire County Council 1991:167). The team deplored the lack of proper and independent professional input and its report acts as a warning to services for adults and children with disabilities which may also seek to justify or dress up poor practice in therapeutic jargon.

The law however, whether for children or adults, may make no provision for genuine emergencies or provide guidance about what is appropriate or permitted. Lyon (1994)

101

commented on the absence of any specific reference to the needs of children with severe behaviour problems and intellectual disabilities in the United Kingdom's 1989 Children Act, a major piece of legislation on children's rights and protection. She extracted some guidance from codes of practice attached to Mental Health Legislation about seclusion but when considering what might be acceptable forms of restraint she concludes that *"the case law is silent as to permissible forms of restraint"* (Lyon 1994:91). This silence came about because the difficult decisions and dilemmas which arise in the context of caring for children with such intense needs had not been envisaged.

New legislation in Norway regulates the use of force and coercion by public authorities in relation to certain people with intellectual disabilities and challenging behaviour. The scope of this legislation is to avoid "significant harm in a situation of actual danger". This includes the use of instruments for electronic tagging and surveillance to give an alarm or warning and elements of coercion in behaviour modification programmes. Measures are defined as coercive when the recipient objects to, or resists them or when they are particularly intrusive. The Act's intention is to regulate the use of force and this is made clear in its title "The rights of, and restrictions on, and control of, the use of coercion and force on certain mentally retarded persons."

The law was initially passed for a period of 3 years, later extended to 5 years at which point it will be reviewed in the light of an evaluation. The framework set out in the legislation would only authorise coercive or intrusive interventions if:

- alternative measures had been tried and failed;

- the amount of force to be used was proportional to the purpose to be achieved and should not exceed what is necessary to achieve this goal;

- procedural clearance was sought in advance of any intervention.

The following case study illustrates how this legislation might plug a gap in protection for the most vulnerable people with disabilities.

The case refers to an autistic and mentally retarded woman in a small town in Norway who had a long history of self-injurious behaviour. More than 5000 self-injuring incidents had been registered in just one day. She had blinded herself in one eye, damaged the other, seriously injured her ears and heels and damaged her knees, and she wore a helmet to avoid further head and brain injuries. She weighed only 34 kilos, and there was an immediate danger that she might actually die of under-nourishment. She was kept on rather heavy medication to control the worst outbursts of self-injury.

The municipality finally contacted a psychologist with considerable experience in working with these kinds of problems. He devised a training programme designed to eliminate – or at least significantly reduce – the self-injurious behaviour, teach her basic language functions (she lacked a properly functioning language) and tackle her eating (and sleeping) problems. There were no particular rules or regulations directly relevant to such treatment programmes under the old law, neither as regards procedure nor legality. Use of force would have to be judged according to the rules regarding self-defence and necessity as stated in the penal code.

The training programmes involved many things, among them two controversial items, which were used to break off a sequence of self-injuring behaviour. One was called "guided walk" which meant that two employees held the woman's arms behind her back and walked fast – or ran – with her in a zigzag pattern to avoid her throwing herself down on her knees or otherwise hurting herself. These exercises could go on for as long as 20 minutes and be repeated up to 20 times a day. The other was a kind of "sit-up", which meant that she would be placed on a chair with her head towards the floor and then would have to raise herself up to a sitting position. This procedure was used during meals, if she injured herself or otherwise behaved in a way that was not compatible with eating.

The case actually came to be heard before the court under employment law because one nurse objected to this treatment and refused to participate in it; her refusal led to a dispute with the municipality in their role as her employer.

Under the old system there would have been no specific legal mechanism for scrutinising this treatment programme. Under the new legislation (chapter 6A) a case like this would be handled along the following lines: The municipality would have to present its proposal for treatment to the County Governor for approval. Before the County Governor could make a decision, various parties would be heard (within a week), such as relatives, guardian or assistant guardian (one of whom is compulsory in these cases) and the County municipal specialist service for the mentally retarded. The County Governor's decision could later be appealed to an administrative court on the County municipal level and further to the ordinary courts, beginning with the municipality courts. In order to gain the County Governor's approval, the treatment would need to be shown to be professionally and ethically justifiable. Less intrusive methods should have been tried (or sufficient reasons given as to why this had not been done). The treatment would have to be *proportional to* the purpose to be achieved (in this case to save the woman's life and reduce or eliminate her self-injuring behaviour), and the treatment the least intrusive available; the coercive element of the intervention must not go further than necessary. In addition the treatment must comply with further regulations that among other things state that treatment methods causing physical and/or psychical harm or significant physical or psychical strain are not allowed. If approved, the actual treatment would then be subject to review by the County Governor.

There is clearly a valid debate about whether it is more effective to acknowledge a need for physical intervention or aversive programmes in some instances and strictly limit their application or to endorse a complete "ban" which offers no guidance to those staff who find themselves acting in an emergency. In the United Kingdom a policy document on physical interventions (Harris et al. 1996) aimed to achieve similar ends through operational guidance to staff (see section 6) but this has been superseded by statutory guidance which is in draft form at the time of writing. The voluntary code set out a process for service providers to work through in relation to every individual who might demand a physical or containing response to difficult behaviour. It can be referenced in contracts between service providers and local authorities but does not currently have any legal basis.

Conversely people with behavioural problems are the most likely to be on the receiving end of physical interventions, especially where their challenging behaviour is associated with significant and pervasive intellectual disabilities and/or is has a neurological basis. Supporting the development of staff skills in behaviour analysis and behavioural treatment is the only way to ensure that this group of people with disabilities are managed in such a way that their behaviour does not reach a level to warrant such interventions whether or not these are specified in law.

4.4. Facilitating access to justice and redress

Accessing justice is a complex process and there are many barriers to appropriate and successful prosecution, in theory and in practice. Access may require specific support to be made available to disabled individuals to help them consider the pros and cons of reporting wrongs to the police. Police officers and lawyers working within the criminal justice system also need expert advice. This should help them provide an equitable service to disabled children and adults and assistance to compensate for any specific impairments or additional vulnerability.

One model is that of the Swiss Juris Conseil Junior, an association set up under the aegis of the Geneva Bar which regroups barristers and social actors and two instructors from the Geneva Youth Health Service. Its primary aim is to make sure all minors have unconditional access to the legal and judicial system, regardless in particular of their social background, by granting them immediate legal aid in the spirit of the 1989 Convention on the rights of the Child. Juris Conseil Junior offers a confidential help line which offers free advice and, if a case is to be opened, the financial arrangements are made individually to make sure that everyone has access.

Specific adaptations are made for disabled children and young adults (example submitted by the Swiss delegation).

In the United Kingdom an independent voluntary organisation (VOICE United Kingdom) offers support to people with learning disabilities, family members and staff around sexual abuse, with a specific emphasis on supporting them through any court action. The organisation has also campaigned around changing the law and making adaptations to courtroom practice and has been instrumental in bringing about a review of courtroom practice for all vulnerable and intimidated witnesses (Home Office 1998). This organisation was founded by a parent whose daughter was sexually abused by a care worker. The parent had a considerable struggle to ensure that the worker was brought to justice. Relatives' groups have also been formed where a number of individuals have been affected by abuse in a residential home or institution and their campaigns have highlighted departures from normal practice where cases involve disabled children or adults. For example in France a case involving the kidnapping, sexual abuse and murder of seven mentally handicapped young women between 1977 and 1979 was not properly prosecuted until a relatives' group was formed in 1996. The outrage of these families was not only directed at an anomaly of the law which would allow the perpetrator to walk free because of the length of time which has passed since the murders but also at

> *"the shocking lack of concern it has revealed on the part of the social services. The police were never officially informed of the girls' disappearances ... " (Henley 2000b:19).*

4.4.1. Courtroom practice

When people with disabilities have been wronged they are often disregarded by the very systems which should uphold their rights. Awareness needs to be raised amongst law enforcement agencies to counter the view that people with disabilities are/can be neither worthy victims or reliable witnesses. Practices embedded in years of tradition must be countered if institution-wide biases are to be stopped.

Equitable access to redress through the criminal justice system is central to the broader campaign being conducted by people with disabilities and their organisations against all forms of discrimination and exclusion. The European Disability Forum (1999a:15) note that:

"in many countries access to justice for people with disabilities is often restricted by problems relating to both the physical and social accessibility of the courts, statutory provisions on evidence, legal procedures and the lack of willingness on the part of magistrates to adapt to the individual differences which result from handicap."

Progress has been made in relation to children's evidence in many member states. In inquisitorial systems (for example France and the Netherlands) children's statements used to be admitted in written form after their initial interview but France has recently moved towards video-recorded interviews in some cases. In accusatorial systems the requirement for live, oral evidence has had to be adapted to allow for the use of videotaped interviews and cross examination via video links (Spencer 1997). For example in the United Kingdom guidance on video interviewing of children's evidence has been in place since 1992 and will shortly be revised and extended to vulnerable adults after considerable evaluation (Westcott & Jones 1997).

In the United Kingdom initial caution about the usefulness of videotaped evidence has largely evaporated (Davies & Wilson 1997:10) with the exception of defence barristers who continue to argue for live cross-examination in court. All the other professional groups involved have welcomed the reduction of stress for children giving evidence this way. The Memorandum sought both to enable good practice by allowing service providers latitude to tailor methods of enquiry to the individual child and to prescribe minimum standards which legitimate the admission of the child's evidence in court. This inevitably produces conflicts. Wade and Westcott (1997:60) argued that interviews held too soon <u>for the child</u> were:

"premised on disclosure as an event rather than a dynamic process through which children move" and tended to produce

107

"tentative and incomplete evidence which may later be used to undermine a child capable of providing credible court testimony".

For a detailed analysis of how children's evidence is admitted into court across member states see Spencer (1997).

Moreover there is a need to dovetail the interview with other investigative activities and not burden a child or vulnerable adult's testimony by allowing it to be the sole or primary source of evidence (Brown et al. 1996). Practice in interviewing is only one strand in the work of evidence gathering and detection. Critics have argued that the Memorandum attempts to place too much weight on the child's evidence and that the emphasis should switch towards investigating adults rather than questioning children, and being more proactive in seeking out other sources of evidence. Moves toward more proactive investigation and evidence gathering might be particularly appropriate to the needs of disabled children and adults whose accounts may sometimes be more difficult to obtain.

Related measures included in "Speaking up for Justice" – a Home Office consultation document on Vulnerable and Intimidated Witnesses – included:

- early identification of vulnerability by police and other agencies;
- facilitating access to specialist advice and assistance in interviewing;
- guidance on pre-trial support;
- changes in courtroom practice.

These elements have formed the core of an extensive implementation programme (Home Office 1999).

4.4.2. Consistent sentencing

There is evidence across member states of anomalies in sentencing where crimes involve people with disabilities. For example where there are specific sexual offences applying to people with intellectual disabilities these may carry lesser penalties to their generic equivalents (e.g. rape). In other contexts the legal code is underlined in relation to children or vulnerable adults by stricter penalties especially for sexual offences against children and/or to be applied to those who have committed their offences while in a position of trust or authority. Vulnerable *adults* may not be included in these provisions. As Stanko (2000:250) remarks:

> *"In political rhetoric perhaps victims of violence are ... all 'innocent' and in need of protection. In reality, many differences and circumstances divide victims and contribute to whether and how the state through its criminal justice apparatus intervenes ... In many cases the burden of responsibility to initiate intervention and then to be steadfastly committed to seeing this intervention through is displaced onto the individuals."*

Vulnerability may not always be apparent in victims especially where they come from stigmatised or stereotyped communities or groups. Hence people with mental health, drug or alcohol problems tend to be characterised as "dangerous" instead of "vulnerable", while people with certain physical disabilities are treated as if they are more frail and less able to take care of themselves than they actually are.

A mixed picture emerges from member states: in the Netherlands sentencing is the same whether or not a victim is disabled but there is an additional offence where sexual acts are committed against someone with a severe physical or intellectual disability and who is thereby unable to give their consent even if it does not involve force or violence. In other words the principle here is that usually when sex occurs without force there is a presumption that it is consenting but if the person is deemed not to be able to give their own it is assumed that the acts have taken place against the person's will. A similar offence exists in United Kingdom legislation. Sexual offence legislation in Luxembourg also prescribes additional penalties where a sexual assault or rape is carried out by someone in a position of influence or authority, or where their victim is under 14. In Spain and Slovenia disability can be treated as an aggravating circumstance when sentencing offenders. Moreover Spanish law makes it clear that where crimes are motivated by racism, anti-Semitism, religious, sexual or disablist discrimination, these will be regarded as aggravating circumstances. In Italy, the Law 269/98 (Norms against the exploitation of children in prostitution, pornography and sex tourism; article 6) stipulates additional penalties to offenders when the victim is physically or mentally disabled.

4.5. Summary

This chapter has reviewed a number of layers of legal protection for people with disabilities. Each will be present in different forms in the legal codes of member states. The following questions provide a template for briefly auditing this provision.

Defining abuse against people with disabilities

• Are disabled children and adults equitably protected by generic laws which refer to property crime (theft, fraud, burglary) and crime against the person (assault, rape, sexual assault, murder)?

• Do investigative activities and sentencing policies take vulnerability into account and give clear signals that crime against vulnerable children and adults will be taken seriously?

• Do statutes which define sexual assaults and rape make specific reference to people who do not have capacity to consent?

• Are there specific offences which define sexual acts between professional carers/service providers and those they care for as exploitative in situations where individual people with disabilities may be unable to resist or get away from pressure or coercion?

• Do laws define incest as a criminal act to children and to adults? Are people with disabilities implicitly or explicitly included within these laws?

110

- Is it clear that the general criminal code is applicable to all children and adults including those who live in residential homes, hospitals or other secure or controlled settings?

- Are disabled adults (excepting those who lack capacity) accorded adult status and rights to enter into binding contracts, enter/leave relationships, live independently from their parents?

Preventative mechanisms

Does the legal system:

- include anti-discrimination legislation in relation to people with disabilities in housing employment, health-care and the provision of goods and services;

- identify those people who do not have capacity to make certain (well-defined) decisions for themselves and /or manage their financial affairs and provide a system for designating someone to act on their behalf and review such appointments;

- require staff who work with disabled children and vulnerable adults to be screened to see if they have been previously convicted of relevant offences;

- review and evaluate grounds for detention and or any element of compulsory treatment with provision for appeal and independent advocacy;

- stipulate how the rights of those who are compulsorily detained can be safeguarded and independently scrutinized;

- provide judicial review of any decision to sterilise a disabled person who lacks capacity to make their own decision about such an irreversible intervention;

- insist on specific safeguards for people with disabilities in relation to any end-of-life decisions such as a "do not resuscitate" determination or physician-assisted suicide in any countries where this has been legalized;

111

- provide additional support to anyone with a disability who is being interviewed as a potential suspect in relation to a criminal act?

Facilitate access to legal system

- Are cases in which a disabled person has been the victim of a crime brought to court in an equivalent way to those cases which involve other citizens?

- Are cases in which disabled persons are represented, as victim, witnesses or defendant, heard in courtrooms which make available:

  - wheelchair access;

  - interpretation in sign language, alternative communication systems, minority languages;

  - provision for video linked evidence from children and or vulnerable adults;

  - arrangements to ensure that unnecessary repeat interviews and hearings are avoided;

  - facility for cross examination via video link;

  - informal atmosphere for children or adults who might otherwise be intimidated;

  - questioning in a manner and in language which matches the ability and understanding of any disabled person involved;

  - screens so that vulnerable witnesses or victim do not have to face the accused person?

- Is expert evidence and specialized psychological assessment allowed into court proceedings to prevent a disabled person's truthfulness being wrongfully impugned (see Yuille 1988)?

- Are people with disabilities who are convicted of crimes diverted to the secure mental health system where this is appropriate?

- Are people with disabilities who are held in prison or other secure settings assured that their special needs are taken into account including their need to be protected from other inmates; access to any special equipment or and provision of appropriate and equivalent health care?

Where people with disabilities come into contact with the criminal justice system as defendants or offenders it is important that their mental, physical or intellectual disabilities are not allowed to disadvantage or deny them proper advocacy and, if they are convicted, equitable treatment.

Equitable redress

Clearly people with disabilities are entitled both to be treated equitably in law whether they are victims of crime, witnesses or defendants *and* they are also entitled to any extra assistance that they need in order to access proper justice on their own behalf and on behalf of others.

Does the law deliver redress to people with disabilities who are victims of crime, discrimination or wrongful action in ways which signal that it:

- values the lives of people with disabilities equitably when damages or compensation is awarded;
- prescribes equivalent penalties which signal the value attached to people with disabilities and places a high priority on their protection?

These aspirations for equitable access to justice are consistent with the disability specific non-discrimination directive of the European Union (European Disability Forum (EDF) 1999b).

113

5. WORKING TO ACHIEVE GOOD PRACTICE

5.1. Models of prevention

This chapter provides examples of work that is being done to strengthen protection for individuals both within specific social care agencies and in a broader social context. All the parties to this report agree that "prevention" is of paramount importance but in order to see how this broad range of initiatives fit together it is necessary to produce a conceptual map. Vettenburg (Dubet & Vettenburg 1999:43) commented that:

> *"Like 'violence', 'prevention' is a term which has many connotations and therefore needs to be described and defined clearly".*

A concern with prevention arises in the context of crime, illness and (more controversially) disability and presupposes that these events/conditions are both undesirable and avoidable. Most pragmatists seek to minimise risks while recognising that interventions will also be needed to address those situations where primary prevention has not been possible.

Several theoretical models have been developed. Many social theorists borrow from health promotion the model of primary, secondary and tertiary prevention. This model categorises interventions in terms of different stages:

• at the primary stage which prevents abuse from happening at all;

• at a secondary stage to ensure that abuse is promptly identified and referred to appropriate agencies who will intervene to stop it recurring and;

• at the tertiary stage to treat individuals who have been abused and help them to recover without sustaining long-term problems related to trauma and distress.

Hardiker, Exton and Barker (1995) analysed social policy and the role of the state in relation to the prevention of child abuse – mapping involvement at different stages and at different levels and arguing that governments which regarded their role as residual would become involved at a later stage and only with individuals who had already been damaged. Conversely those which embraced a broader commitment would become involved before harm had been done and attempt to influence attitudes across the whole population in order to prevent abuse from occurring in the first place.

Vettenburg (Dubet & Vettenburg1999) addressed prevention in a comparable Council of Europe document on prevention of violence in schools: her construction has also been helpful to us in bringing together initiatives which address different parts of the system at different stages in the aetiology of the problem. She noted four distinct "prototypes" in the range of preventative strategies submitted (adapted from Dubet & Vettenburg 1999):

- situational prevention, that is attending to the environments in which abuse may take place through for example the design of establishments or staff supervision;

- punitive prevention, where by attending to detection, prosecution and appropriately serious punishment sets up a sufficient deterrent;

- treatment-based prevention which conceptualises abuse as a consequence of individual or family dysfunction or prior victimisation of the perpetrator;

- social prevention, which deals with the problem in the broader social context, for example by addressing specific manifestations of abuse against a backdrop of widespread discrimination against people with disabilities.

Hence she also describes preventative strategies in terms of *stages* and *levels* but adds a third dimension which explores the *nature* or *orientation* of the intervention in terms of whether it is primarily defensive or offensive; we might also refer to these as reactive or proactive.

In relation to abuse a *defensive (reactive)* strategy would be one which seeks to avert danger, for example through screening out unsuitable staff, whereas an offensive (proactive) strategy will tackle risks by promoting positives through for example enhancing user involvement, improving key areas of practice or implementing quality assurance programmes. An overly defensive approach will end up cutting across important competing principles such as fostering autonomy or increasing openness and integration. Vettenburg argues that in her field, a set of preferred options have emerged which consist of primary prevention, at a structural level and with a proactive orientation.

Our aim in this chapter is to set out as strongly as possible the argument that governments should invest in prevention and that they should give this commitment a high profile.

5.1.1. Taking action at all levels

The working group and those bodies they consulted have been at one in advocating that action is needed at all these levels to assure proper protection and redress on behalf of people with disabilities across member States. The European Disability Forum (EDF) (1999a) have voiced the following priorities in taking action against abuse:

- that abuses be seen in the context of more widespread discrimination against people with disabilities;
- that these should be conceptualised as a basic human rights issue;
- that a sounder knowledge base needs to be built up through the collection of more reliable information and the introduction of more sensitive systems to encourage reporting and advocacy and
- that member states take holistic and systematic steps to challenge all abuse and mistreatment as a matter of principle and urgency.

This chapter documents examples of distinct elements within such a "holistic and systematic" strategy. Submissions from

117

member states and NGOs described a range of initiatives including:

- campaigns to raise public awareness;
- educational initiatives such as sex education and self-defence classes for disabled children, young people and adults;
- policy documents to guide interagency working;
- professional training and support;
- improved investigation to bring perpetrators to justice;
- monitoring and inspection of institutional settings (especially for sexual violence);
- complaints procedures;
- user involvement;
- measures to facilitate access to courts and legal advocacy;
- counselling services for people with disabilities and their families;
- treatment /interventions for potential perpetrators;
- campaigning groups and NGOs with a specific remit to address issues of abuse of people with disabilities;
- programmes concerning the recruitment and supervision of volunteers;
- training and accreditation of professional groups working with people with disabilities;
- arrangements for independent inspection and scrutiny of institutions and day centres.

A similar range of initiatives has been reported in North America and in relation to other client groups. Wolf and Pillimer (1994) described four models of good practice in relation to elder abuse, a multidisciplinary case conference team, a volunteer advocacy programme, a victim support group and a master's degree in adult protection for social workers

These initiatives represent action designed both to prevent abuse and to provide an adequate response once it has been identified. We have documented interventions at different *levels* (individual, organisational and political) and by different *agencies,* with a focus ranging from the interaction between individual people with disabilities and their carers to the training of judges in how to evaluate evidence from people with communication impairments (see Directorate General III – Social Cohesion 2000). None of these stands alone, nor can they be seen as entirely discrete. Each programme will have knock-on effects, for example better identification and more effective sanctions (secondary prevention) may in turn act as a sufficient deterrent to prevent abuse from taking place at all (primary prevention) and programmes which help people with disabilities to become more assertive may allow people with disabilities to challenge potential abusers and prevent abuse from occurring (primary prevention) or enable individuals to challenge violations of their human rights retrospectively through the courts and make a good recovery (tertiary prevention).

Examples of a range of interventions at different levels are included in the following table and details of several initiatives are set out.

5.1.2. A range of interventions

Focus	Level	Primary	Secondary	Tertiary
Individual		Self-help campaigns such as the "Keep children safe" campaign pioneered by Kidscape in the United Kingdom which educate children about "good and bad" touch; the French/Belgian initiative "La violence, parlons-on"; self-defence workshops for disabled women co-ordinated by Lydia Zijdel (The Netherlands).	User-friendly leaflets in a range of accessible formats spelling out for people with disabilities what their rights are and how to make a complaint.	Equitable and respectful media coverage of cases in which victim is a disabled person.
Service providers and commissioners		Staff training and guidance on difficult areas of practice especially challenging behaviour, control and restraint and sexuality. Screening of staff who are going to work with disabled children or adults before they begin work. Bodies to oversee professional registration and regulation.	Training on how to recognise abuse and how to make referrals evidenced by detailed policies and procedures within and between agencies. Formal guidance about how vulnerable children and adults who are witnesses or victims can be interviewed and give their evidence in court.	Debriefing after incidents. Formal inquiries to ensure lessons are learned and fed back into practice. Poor homes closed down where improvements not likely within given time-scale. Some specialised services with expertise in working with abused people.

	Regulation of settings and regular inspection to raise standards.	Training for mainstream agencies working with abused people, e.g. rape crisis, women's refuges, or victim support, in how to make their services accessible to people with disabilities.
Government and community	Public information campaigns to explain what constitutes abuse and advertise points for referral. Help lines to offer advice to carers and staff. Structural support for whistle-blowers (Pilgrim 1995) in the form of good employment protection, protection through trades unions and professional associations. Links across mainstream agencies such as social services, health, police and criminal justice systems.	High level review of cases to develop policy with integral safeguards. Workforce planning and review of training needs. Mechanisms for tracking abusive staff as they move across county, regional and national borders. New legislation where this is needed. Responsible media coverage which balances a recognition of vulnerability with a respect for people with disabilities as citizens and not victims.
	Campaigns to counter stereotypes and negative images of people with disabilities' lives. Integration and anti-discrimination campaigns which highlight the human rights of people with disabilities and clarify when boundaries have been crossed. Media campaigns which show people how to communicate and interact with people who have different impairments. Adequate funding and accountable use of resources on behalf of people with disabilities and agencies which exist to serve them.	

121

5.2. Primary prevention

5.2.1. At individual level

One strategy for the prevention of sexual abuse of children and adults with intellectual and communication disabilities has been skilled sex education and this has been acknowledged, for example, in the United Kingdom, the Netherlands, Norway and Switzerland. Materials are available in several countries (see for example McCarthy & Thompson 1997; Delville & Mercier 1997; Delville, Mercier & Merlin 2000; Belie, Ivens, Lesseliers & Hove 2000) many of which have adapted mainstream curricula for children and adults with special educational needs. Other materials have been directed at staff to help them address the needs of specific groups such as those with profound handicaps (Down & Craft 1997), or intellectually disabled sex offenders (Thompson & Brown 1998; Terstegen, Hoekman & Bergh 1998) and staff training modules of two or more days are offered by agencies in a number of member states. In Switzerland, the French-speaking and international Association on Sexuality and Physical Disability (SEHP) provides training to care professionals and educational staff as well as persons with physical disabilities in the form of sessions which are always given jointly by a specialised sex educator and a person with the disability concerned who is already well aware of the subject.

The involvement of parents and professionals and the information about issues related to sexuality that can be given to them are considered essential. In fact, all these persons are "third parties" who take part in supporting the everyday life of the disabled person and especially in situations of intimacy. Agthe Diserens and Vatré (2000a), two specialised sex educators, have designed a programme for awareness raising and training of these parental and educational partners. The programme – *Du Coeur au Corps, formons-nous, puis ... formons-les!* – received the Swiss Prize 2001 for Remedial Education. It covers themes such as love, genital organs, contraception, sterilisation, sorrow for the loss of a child, sexual abuse, intimity, marriage and celibacy (note of Swiss delegation).

Signing (for deaf children and adults see Kennedy in ABCD pack) and pictorial systems such as Bliss need to be adapted to include body parts and terms for unpleasant acts so that children can report mistreatment. For example boards may not have any words for "hit" or "smack" or for private body parts. Attention to communication aids may greatly strengthen children's rights and act as a deterrent to abuse. One case of serial sexual abuse at a special residential school for frail and severely disabled children in the United Kingdom was uncovered by painstaking interviews using augmented communication boards and this approach has since been developed into a school-wide "Know your rights" campaign for both students and staff as recorded in Marchant & Page (1992).

The Italian Society for children and adults with Down syndrome has introduced programmes of "education in self reliance", which are conducted in single sex groups, and use a variety of films, slides, and videos to stimulate questions and discussion on topics such as falling in love, affection, reactions to unwanted sexual advances, what it means to have Down syndrome etc. Another joint project (Delville, Mercier & Merlin 2000) previously referred to, has been based on collaboration between two sex education specialists from Switzerland and the Psychology Department of the Faculty for Medicine at the University of Namur consisting of a special curriculum on love life and sexuality for people with intellectual disabilities and an ethical guide for staff. A service based at the Horizon Trust in Hertfordshire, United Kingdom (CONSENT) combines individual programmes of assessment, counselling and education with staff development and training has also been developed alongside an innovative service which provides assessment for people with intellectual disabilities who are referred as a result of sexual offending behaviour (RESPOND). Clearly it is necessary to provide resources to allow these centres of excellence to develop and to cross–fertilise their direct treatment and staff training programmes.

In Luxembourg, the United Kingdom and the Netherlands assertiveness and self-defence training for women with intellectual disabilities has raised awareness and self-esteem and provided a space in which abuse can be disclosed. Slovenia has also organised an awareness campaign both to help vulnerable people prevent abuse and also to tell them how to go about reporting any abuses to the police. A Belgian programme entitled "La violence, parlons-en" was adapted for secondary school pupils in the Nord-Pas de Calais region (in France) and developed for use with young people with intellectual disabilities by introducing a series of psychodrama sessions in place of a film. This enabled the young people to tackle the issue of violence and to work though a number of possible responses. An independent sociological evaluation of the programme concluded that

- it helped social workers to see the young people in a more positive light, as they played a very active part in the sessions and made very relevant contributions;
- it had a calming effect on the social and institutional atmosphere in the establishment;
- real communication began to take place both among the young people and between them and the staff;
- young people with disabilities stated that they were prepared to take responsibility for their own violent behaviour and to talk to a responsible adult if they found themselves victims of violence.

While such programmes can help individuals to resist abusive acts and strengthen their resolve to seek help if they are victimised, it is important not to underestimate the skill of determined offenders (especially in the field of sexual abuse) or to slip into a victim–blaming stance towards individuals who have not been able to stand up for their rights in difficult situations.

Other strategies for strengthening individuals have been rooted in the development of alternative service models. It is apparent that abuse thrives in the kind of closed dependency relationships in which people with disabilities are often trapped (Westcott 1993). New models of service which allow individual people with disabilities to manage their own funds and assistance and which favour small group homes over large institutions are preferred for this reason and do make a fundamental difference to the interaction which occurs between individuals and their helpers/carers. User involvement in the running of services not only helps to develop assertiveness and self-confidence in the client group as a means of challenging practices which violate human rights but also provides a source of independent advocacy, and a route through which individuals can make complaints. The Flemish government in Belgium legislated for user participation in the running of residential homes and institutions in 1993. In 1998, the participation of people with disabilities in the running of institutions was made mandatory through the establishement of users' councils in the French-speaking region of Belgium. Estonia has also begun to work towards patient representation. Complaints systems are in operation in both countries. Independent user groups, operating outside any particular service setting strengthen individuals and provide independent scrutiny of services. Two such networks were cited by delegates each of which has successfully raised awareness and strengthened individual people with disabilities.

Example 1

Slovenian Association of disabled students

Students, who have to manage their care and study needs within a fixed budget, formed a group to campaign for resources under the auspices of the University of Llubljana students' organisation in 1996. It has since expanded to become a national association for all students and currently has over 70 members. Their campaigns have included getting more specially adapted accommodation within the university's main housing blocks and improving access, special aids, transport, leisure, sport and training. They have also co-ordinated a public awareness campaign through radio programmes and newspaper articles. Their goals for the future include extending their activities to housing and employment issues facing members after they graduate, building on international links they have established with the Disabled

Student's Association at the University of Cork. A counselling service has already been set up for this purpose.

Example 2

Norwegian disabled women's network

This is a user-led initiative funded by the Norwegian Ministry for Health and Social Affairs in collaboration with Lillehammer College which provides professional support to the network of 100 women all across Norway who communicate through phone calls, newsletters and e-mail. The focus of the network's activity is to promote health improvements and monitor the responses of the health service to women with disabilities. The network also collaborates with women's refuges across Norway and as part of this collaboration they are planning to run a three-year research project on violence against women with disabilities with Ostlandsforskning, a research foundation in Lillehammer. In 1999 the network produced a directory and guide covering a number of key issues including welfare benefits, housing and a separate guide on violence against women with disabilities which is distributed through women's shelters. They have also worked with the refuges to make their premises accessible and their staff welcoming to disabled women. The network supports a more explicitly "gendered" analysis of violence and disability.

A number of these projects illustrate the benefits of close links between academic centres, service providers and user networks. Such collaborations facilitate professional support, systematic evaluation of initiatives and widespread dissemination of good practice.

5.2.2. At service level

In the United Kingdom two NGO's were commissioned in 1993 to write a model policy document for residential services outlining preventative steps in response to research indicating the extent of sexual abuse of people with intellectual disabilities. While it was acknowledged that it was impossible to rule out abuse in any setting, careful strategies for "Lowering the odds" were set out which relied on each individual knowing the extent and limits of their responsibilities (ARC/NAPSAC 1993). One issue highlighted in this report was the need for sound recruitment procedures including screening of potential staff in homes for children and adults with disabilities – possibly through the mechanism of a "good conduct" certificate, police search or registration with a professional body.

Guidance to staff also emerges as an important issue. Although the law provides a framework for making balanced decisions very few cases get to court or are dealt with formally. Everyday oppressions and denials happen without debate or scrutiny and decisions with far reaching implications are often made by staff who may have inadequate training or knowledge about the limits of their legitimate powers. The "rules" and expectations about sharing information between services is also an important issue. Within services, policies and informal guidelines are more likely to shape the behaviour and attitudes of staff than case law. In order to prevent abuse it is necessary to build on positive practices especially in those areas where poor practice can slip over into abuse. Hence services need to develop clear and explicit guidelines to govern the work of staff in relation to:

- sexuality;
- challenging behaviour;
- control and restraint;
- handling money;
- administering medication.

A number of examples of such guidance were submitted by different delegations.

Example 1

Cap Loisirs Foundation, Geneva (Switzerland)

> This organisation offering leisure activities, short and long holidays for disabled persons has produced a charter on "love and sexuality among disabled citizens" which stipulates the rights of people with disabilities and users of holiday camps and other leisure activities to love and sexual life. The staff guidance needed that such relationships take place in the context of mutual respect of all parties is guaranteed by continuous awareness training

127

given to staff and by the means of a code of ethics. The parents and supervisors are required to take note of the conditions stipulated by the charter. This document refers back to the Declaration of Human Rights and the Declaration of General and Particular Rights of Mentally Disabled People. The preparation of this charter is the result of an important partnership between the Cap Loisirs staff, specialized sex educators, parents and tutors as well as directors of institutions.

Example 2

UNAPEI network on sexuality

In 1998 the UNAPEI (Union nationale des associations de parents et amis de personnes handicapées mentales) followed up work on sexuality and AIDS/HIV issues by setting up a working group on ill-treatment. Its aim was to set up a network of relevant persons and bodies including parents and service users. After a period of research and consultation the group produced a policy document setting out a description of the problem, the risks and recommendations. This forms the basis of a strategy to prevent all forms of abuse against children and adults in different settings (including families, institutions, society, medical circles) [UNAPEI 2000].

Example 3

Guidance to staff on physical restraint

A training manual has been produced by the British Institute of Learning Disabilities (BILD) which outlines a process for each service to work through in order to assess and anticipate the needs of people with challenging behaviour who might need to be subjected to physical interventions (control and restraint) in crisis situations. The document works from a very explicit set of values and principles about minimising any force used in such interventions and is predicated on the need for solutions which are individually tailored to the needs and likely problems presented by individuals and not a blanket set of responses to be used across a whole service. Physical interventions are always to be the last resort and to take place against a backdrop of positive approaches and individual treatment. Local procedures using this framework encourage planning in relation to anticipated crises as opposed to ad hoc approaches or emergency responses. The authors advocate a strict "gradient of control" so that incidents are managed using the least force necessary and that any physical intervention ceases as soon as the situation becomes calmer. This approach makes clear that any physical interventions which are necessary to contain a violent incident are not to be used as a cover for punishment or retaliation.

5.2.3 At government and community level

At government and community level it is important that other mainstream projects such as those funded by the EC through its Daphne initiative to address violence against all children, young persons and women should be inclusive of disabled children and adults (note of Italian delegation). The legislative framework needs to be addressed under this heading as does the structure and adequacy of benefit levels and the options available to people with disabilities. Regulation and inspection of professions and services (see Davies & Beach 2000), measures to raise standards through quality assurance and outside scrutiny all have a part to play in bringing about safer services as does the infrastructure which allows for a planned, skilled and well regulated workforce. These structural issues may get downplayed in a model of abuse prevention which relies too heavily on individuals standing up for their own rights or resisting concerted violations.

5.3. Secondary prevention

5.3.1. At individual level

In a survey of people with intellectual disabilities about bullying (Mencap 1999) respondents were asked what would have helped them to cope. Their answers were as follows:

- someone to talk to (70%);
- to know who they could tell about the bullying (58%);
- to know how to make a complaint(48%);
- to know how to report matters to the police (47%).

A number of member states have tackled this dearth of accessible information. The Slovenian authorities have publicised legislation and issued leaflets on how people with disabilities can report crimes to the police. Advocacy agencies such as the Swiss Juris Conseil described above also make it possible for individuals who have been victimised to bring the matter to the attention of the responsible agencies.

5.3.2. At service level

Staff training is the responsibility of individual services but also of governments. At a service level, staff need to be trained to be alert to signals of abuse or abusing but also their training and ongoing supervision must be directed at helping them develop the professional skills and personal maturity to avoid abusing those in their care (AEP 2000:3). Turk and Brown (1993) found that disclosure was the most frequent trigger to sexual abuse referrals of intellectually disabled adults. Staff training should focus on how to listen and what to do in the immediate aftermath of a disclosure: on how far to seek supportive information from the person, how to deal with requests to keep the matter confidential and how to record the disclosure in a way which leaves open the possibility of taking legal action. A fundamental issue is to help staff explore their own values and practice and to set for themselves a "line" beyond which they would report concerns about the behaviour of colleagues or family members. The AIMS materials (1998) provide exercises and scenarios to help staff groups reach this kind of shared consensus about the threshold of acceptable practice in relation to different client groups and types of abuse.

Working together across agency and professional divides is a key to helpful responses for both adults and children. In Estonia doctors are required to report signs of violence against patients to the police. In the Netherlands victims may report either to the police or to local authorities and the police draw up a statement, which is then used as the basis of an official report and further decision making. A "pool of experts" is available to help them interview disabled persons in the course of their investigations. In the United Kingdom, social services departments take the lead in co-ordinating an investigation and hold the primary responsibility for deciding on protection, support and treatment for the victim. It might be that support is a more appropriate response to an abuser than sanctions in which case social care agencies provide this. Where necessary the police direct the prosecution process and the inspection unit independently manages the regulatory function, which might lead to an establishment being closed down. The Netherlands has a similar inspection system with mandatory reporting of incidents: the manner in which an agency responds to complaints and concerns provides important clues as to its commitment to quality. Inspectorates also set minimum standards: in the Netherlands these are codified in the 1996 Act governing the "Quality of Care in Institutions" and institutions are required to draw up internal policies to prevent sexual abuse. A model policy might include the following components:

- personnel policy;
- client policy;
- guidelines for care;
- sexual awareness information;
- pointers for prevention of sexual assaults;
- in-house expertise;
- plan for life-long learning;
- profile, tasks and responsibilities of advocates;
- plan for dealing with disclosures;
- example of a complaints procedure.

Professional regulation operates in addition to the regulation of establishments and settings and individual professionals who have been found responsible for abusive incidents may be subject to disciplinary proceedings and/or be prevented from working in a professional capacity with children or vulnerable adults again.

Service workers need to know when, how and to whom they should report concerns, and in what circumstances they should override their usual rules about confidentiality. It is not always clear how far providers of service can be trusted to manage any subsequent investigations without risking con-

131

flicts of interest nor when they can or should involve the police. In countries or areas of work where services are predominantly provided by statutory agencies the independence of inspection and regulatory bodies is important. Conversely when care is provided by private agencies or NGO's, strong oversight from statutory funding bodies or regulators is necessary. What matters is that there are independent checks and balances and a variety of routes through which complaints can be routed. One researcher looking into responses to crime and people with intellectual disabilities used the analogy of a "web" as the strongest model for these safeguards as opposed to a "chain" in which there could easily be a weak link (Williams 1995). In the Netherlands some institutions have a "report team" which investigates a complaint internally and then reports on to the police.

Policy documents are beginning to be drawn up at national, local and agency levels in several member states. These policies aim to fulfill a number of functions:

- to clarify the definition of abuse and heighten awareness;
- to set out what workers have to do when faced with concerns about abuse or disclosures;
- to establish routes for referral and arrangements for joint input to investigations and decision making;
- to set out the situations in which information that might otherwise be confidential could, and should, be shared across agency and professional boundaries;
- to clarify in which circumstances and for which individuals it is justifiable to intervene in families in order to uphold the vulnerable adult's or child's human rights while striking a proper balance between these rights and the family's right to privacy;
- to define in what circumstances a police or other official inquiry can and should be instigated when a vulnerable victim has not, or is not in the position to, give his or her consent or make a formal statement;
- to maximise the extent to which people with disabilities can make their own decisions about the support and protection

they need in the aftermath of abuse without jeopardising action taken against perpetrators;

- to ensure that abusers who might be a risk to other vulnerable adults or children are prevented from working in social care agencies with them or otherwise gaining access to them in future;

- to feed back into services those lessons which have been learned about how to enhance the quality of provision for disabled children and adults and build sensitive safeguards routinely into practice.

Formal complaints systems, operating locally or as part of statutory provisions, are in operation in a number of member states and although they have the advantage of ensuring that once a complaint is made it must receive attention and be followed through, there are still major barriers to reporting and justifiable fears of reprisals or unfair treatment in the wake of making a complaint particularly if the person against whom the complaint is made continues to work in a service used by the complainant. The Spanish delegation submitted a detailed example under this heading which illustrates how a complaints system works at local level operating within central government guidance.

Example 1

Complaints and Suggestions book in Spanish services

There is a basic statute for all residential centres for people with disabilities, laying down rights and duties, and arrangements for user participation through a user's council, governing bodies, assemblies, sanctions and disciplinary measures. Each centre has "in-house rules", "list of services" dispensed by the centre and an official "complaints and suggestions book" available in the information room and help is available to assist individuals to file a complaint. The user keeps one copy, a second is sent to the head of the unit and a third to the general inspectorate at the ministry. Anonymous complaints and suggestions are also accepted and acted upon. The provincial director, within 20 working days, informs the service manager and seeks an explanation and details of any action taken to resolve the complaint; this is then kept on the file. A quarterly summary is drawn up with the aim of informing improvements in the services available (Defensor del Pueblo 1996). The following case study illustrates how the complaints system works in practice – Mr A., a disabled person living in a residential centre, received a visit from his friends but shortly after arriving the visit was cut short by a maintenance officer from the centre who threatened the visitors and asked them to leave the room, although they had official authorisation to be there. This was reported through the complaints book and after an investigation the worker was given a warning for his conduct.

5.3.3. At government and community level

The Council of Europe has issued a series of recommendations in relation to the abuse of all children (Committee of Ministers of the Council of Europe 1993). These recommendations provide a model to illustrate the range of measures that need to be adapted to meet the needs of children and adults with disabilities. Central government guidance is needed to underpin policy and procedures within services and to create an interlocking system of independent "watchdog" arrangements, including the regulation of settings and professions. In Italy, this work is managed by a National Committee of Coordination which acts on behalf of all children.

Example 1

Arrangements for inspection and regulation in France

A government circular dated 5 May 1998 urged all relevant local agencies to identify incidents of abuse against minors [arrangements for disabled/ vulnerable adults have not yet been provided] in educational and social institutions and subsequently issued guidance in the form of a protocol for crisis management in institutions where abuse or violence had occurred, designed to ensure the safety of individuals and to prevent recurrence. As in the United Kingdom, a report of violence would immediately trigger an inspection whose remit includes:

• not to seek proof of guilt but to ensure that the persons in care are not in danger and that the institution is capable of continuing to care for them;

- premises including health and safety arrangements and lay-out of communal areas;
- staff qualifications and numbers and the actual level of staff on duty;
- rules on professional practice and arrangements for monitoring their observance;
- the attitude of the institution's staff to those in their care;
- the employees' perceptions of their work and of the people they care for;
- the medical and psychological care actually provided;
- the effectiveness and relevance of the guidance available to carers;
- the observance of employment regulations [see Ministère de l'emploi et de la solidarité 1999].

If the inspector believes that an offence has been committed, it is their responsibility to report it straight to the police and they are also required to draw up a complete report and put in place provision for follow-up including support for all concerned, removal of any perpetrator, any required changes in the institution's structures or practices for the future and in exceptional circumstances closure. Inspection teams have unrestricted access to observe, visit and ask questions. Broadly speaking, these arrangements parallel those in the United Kingdom, which has an added emphasis on multi-agency working to produce collaboration during any investigation. The aim of this is to avoid repeated interviews of witnesses and victims and to ensure that evidence gathered to support a prosecution can also be made available to those agencies which are responsible for regulating services, taking disciplinary action against employees and providing therapy to individuals who have been harmed.

Example 2

A national training initiative in Portugal

In order to promote special training in the areas of abuse and violence against people with disabilities, a national tertiary educational institute (Instituto Superior de Psicologia Aplicada in Lisbon), responsible for the training of rehabilitation specialists across all disciplines, has recently introduced a 2-level module into the academic curriculum. These modules have been implemented at both pre- and post-graduate levels for students and for professionals seeking to upgrade their qualifications.

Responding to abuse of disabled children and adults requires action by all relevant agencies not only those who have a particular responsibility for people with disabilities and their services. Most agencies of government will have a role to play and corresponding training and information needs to equip them. Governments need to take a lead in setting up partnership arrangements and clarifying responsibilities and channels of communication in relation to both children and adults. Local policies should operate within a mandatory national and local framework.

Example 3

United Kingdom guidance on multi-agency working

A document in the United Kingdom called "Working together" has mandated shared approaches to work on child protection since 1989 and a new document "No secrets" (Department of Health 2000) mirrored by the Welsh Office's "In safe hands" plug the gap for disabled adults. This document attempts to build bridges between these parallel systems by appointing one agency (social services) to take a co-ordinating role locally. The guidance is legally binding on local authorities who are required to make provision for joint working between police, regulators, health and social care professionals in the interests of children and vulnerable adults. It suggests arrangements for clarifying roles and responsibilities and establishing one point for referrals and inquiries. It encourages joint work at a system level in terms of training, pooling resources, mandatory reporting and sharing of information and suggests that agreed procedures are set up for dealing with individual cases. This usually involves a multi-agency assessment or investigation in which information pertaining to serious allegations is to be shared and formal decisions taken and recorded. A similar guidance document has been issued by the French government (Ministère de l'Emploi et de la Solidarité 2000) and by French-speaking Swiss cantons (CCMT 1999).

Example 4

Strategy for service development

The Spanish government submitted a detailed strategy document linking objectives across all agencies including health, mainstreaming in education, economic participation, community integration. Each programme sets out relevant data, strategic objectives and specific courses of action (Ministerio de trabajo y asuntos sociales 1997).

Example 5

National Committee of Co-ordination

In Italy, the Government has set up a National Committee of Co-ordination for the protection of children who have been victims of abuse composed of representatives from relevant government agencies, NGOs and experts working in this field. In addition, the National Plan of Action 2000 – 2001 for the protection of the rights and development of children is aimed at the application and monitoring of the Law 269/98 on the norms against the exploitation of children in prostitution, pornography and sex tourism. Following the Plan of Action, the National Committee of Co-ordination together with the National Observatory for Childhood and Adolescence have issued a co-ordination document with the objective of providing educational programmes regarding the abuse and maltreatment of children as well as obtaining good practices on the issue. This document provides, for example, standardised criteria for classifying and organising statistical data at national and local level and calls for the collection of data on available services and resources. The collected information will be classified and analysed by the National Centre for Documentation and Analysis of Childhood and Adolescence (Florence) which has taken a very active role in this field since its establishment in 1995.

5.3.3.1. Routes through which action may be taken

As we have seen, protective mechanisms are embedded into services at different levels and through different systems. An individual who has been assaulted in a residential home may find the incident dealt with through:

• criminal courts, because a crime has been committed;

137

- regulatory activity against the establishment because standards of care have been breached;

- regulatory activity against a worker who has assaulted them because that worker has breached their professional duties;

- disciplinary action against a worker who is not professionally qualified because their employer wishes to dismiss them;

- a care plan involving another disabled person if they have been assaulted by another service user;

- therapeutic input around their own distress, in addition to or instead of attention being paid to the person/system which is responsible for abusing them;

- a civil case to seek damages/compensation against an individual or corporate body responsible for running their service whose negligence might have caused or contributed to the harm they have suffered.

In theory these mechanisms ought to support each other and provide multiple routes for action to be taken but in practice what has tended to happen is that individual instances can fall between these stand-alone systems. Everyone may think it is someone else's job to take action and no-one is sure which route(s) to take. Several recent inquiries into multiple abuses in the United Kingdom, have demonstrated this confusion and support the case for multi-agency policies which require and enable agencies to work together around abuse issues.

Courtroom procedures should be adapted to be as flexible as is possible without jeopardising natural justice, to allow victims and witnesses who are physically or intellectually disabled or who use alternative or augmented communication systems to participate fully in the quest for justice and redress. Members of the public who will sit on juries or lay panels need to learn about

- services and acceptable practice;

- patterns of abuse and abusing; and

- how to evaluate the testimony of disabled victims and witnesses.

Secondary prevention includes taking action to prevent a recurrence of abuse, whether in the same relationship or setting, or to the same victim but from a different source, or by the same perpetrator to this or further victims. Countries need to harmonise their arrangements for excluding people with certain kinds of convictions from the health/social care workforce. Clearly there is a balance to be drawn which allows for proper rehabilitation of offenders but which protects vulnerable children and adults. Several countries work with "good conduct certificates" or have systems in place which search police records before someone can be employed in this sector, but at present these systems tend to be *ad hoc* and inconsistently applied. A different threshold may be in place in relation to different professional groups or different care sectors. One case which raised these issues in the United Kingdom was of a nurse who had been struck off from his professional register for lesser but related offences but who then raped a women with learning difficulties in the context of his work as an unqualified care assistant (Davies & Beach 2000:226). Moody (1999) explored the same inherent dilemma in relation to volunteering where the stated aims of government to promote social inclusion through encouraging a broad spectrum of citizens to volunteer might be seen to run counter to moves designed to protect vulnerable people from coming into contact with repeat offenders.

5.3.3.2. Confidentiality or secrecy?

Other issues on which government must take a lead include confidentiality which presents difficult dilemmas in these cases. Knowledge of the serial nature of sexual offending in particular has lent urgency to the development of protocols which mandate or at least allow the sharing of information in these cases. A feature of abusive relationships is the enforcement of secrecy through threats and intimidation. Inquiries such as the recent investigations into abuse in children's homes in North Wales often show that fragments of informa-

139

tion are known but not brought together with the result that abuse continues (Waterhouse 2000; Buckinghamshire County Council 1998). Sharing of information within the professional network cuts across this secrecy and ensures that decisions are made as soon as possible with the fullest information available.

Some countries make it mandatory to report child or adult abuse, while others allow more discretion. Estonia is not alone in struggling with this dilemma: at present doctors have a duty to report abuses in the social care (but not health) system but only after they have proof that abuse has taken place. Sharing at this late stage may lead to concerns being suppressed as information known in different parts of the system is not brought together. In the United Kingdom reporting of child protection is mandatory and increasingly this is being reflected in relation to concerns about disabled adults. In the Netherlands it is not compulsory to report either adult or child protection concerns and physicians are bound by the conventions of medical confidentiality. Governments should take a view about how to balance the principle of confidentiality enshrined in data protection legislation with the mandate to share information appropriately and they should act to synchronise the understanding of this responsibility across all the relevant professions which might otherwise work to different standards and with different understandings of abuse.

5.4. Tertiary prevention

This section highlights action which needs to be taken to restore the health and well-being of disabled children and adults who have been abused. It should be noted that previous abuse in childhood or adulthood may contribute to the circumstances which lead individuals to seek services, especially mental health services and that sensitivity to the impact of trauma and abuse should be integral to all assessment and individual planning (Rose, Stratigeas & Peabody 1991). Action will be needed at all levels to inform, develop, fund and evaluate such awareness–raising programmes.

140

5.4.1. At individual level

The Memorandum from the Netherlands highlights the long-term effects of abuse on people who are victims. They note that:

> *"Actual confrontation with violence usually has immense consequences for the person or people involved. An existence which was relatively safe and peaceful until then is brutally shattered and the person feels afraid and unsafe .... People in a vulnerable position whose resilience is limited, in particular, often feel unsafe out-of-doors and at home."*

Research is needed into the effects of abuse on people with disabilities and how these can best be mitigated, including the consequences for mental health of torture, civilian involvement in acts of war, immigration and displacement (see AEP 2000:4). After-effects of abuse are now commonly analysed and understood within the framework of Post Traumatic Stress Disorder which was first added to the American Psychiatric Association's schedule of diagnostic categories in 1994. The term describes a recognised set of mental and physical reactions which can follow trauma including numbness, flashbacks, and hyper-arousal that can sometimes lead to overuse of caffeine or other stimulants. Recognised treatments include medication, cognitive and behavioural psychotherapy techniques. The impact of long-term and/or pervasive abuse is more problematical to analyse within this framework.

Sometimes these consequences can be very difficult to ameliorate, especially when the danger has persisted or the abuse been repeated over time and in the context of a relationship which should have been one of trust and caring. Nor are these effects short-lived. A history of prior abuse may render the person more vulnerable in later life for example by colouring the way they think about risk or diminishing their expectations of future relationships. Abuse may also lead a person to be more vulnerable to repeated victimisation. Evidence suggest that survivors of abuse in childhood are more likely to become the victims of professional abuse in adulthood perhaps because they signal that their boundaries are pregnable or because abusive practitioners sense that they are "comfortable " with violation and even target them in order to "groom" them for abusive relationships (Penfold 1998). A study of young people with disabilities leaving the special school system in Oregon and Nevada (Doren, Bullis & Benz 1996), found that young people who had been victimised at school were six times as likely to be abused again when compared with their peers.

5.4.2. At service level

Most people with disabilities will be best served by accessing those mainstream services which exist to provide long-term support and counselling to all survivors of sexual abuse or domestic violence. Refuges should provide some spaces for women who use wheelchairs and it might be that some specialist refuges are needed to assist women who come from ethnic or linguistic minority communities and/or who those who have special needs. Such access should be negotiated and supported by training on disability issues in these otherwise generic agencies. Disability equality training is usually provided by people with disabilities and provides a structure for challenging discriminatory practice and for challenging a "professional" bias in the way service issues are addressed. In Belgium this training includes a commitment to "de-mystify" disability and in the United Kingdom to disseminate the social model of disability as a basis for service development. The work of the Norwegian women's network has already been noted in this respect. It will be important to know what works if money is to be invested in service provision. Generic victim support schemes are in operation in Portugal, the United Kingdom and other countries.

But some people and communities may need to draw on specialist service provision. A service developed for deaf women and men who have been the victim of personal or sexual violence was developed in Seattle and provides a blueprint for thinking about planning specialist service development in this area (Merkin & Smith 1995). This service (ADWAS) began by monitoring all referrals to learn about the needs of the deaf and deaf-blind community. They were able to then trace shifts in the needs of their service users, noting that at first they served primarily deaf women who had left abusive hearing partners but later served women leaving deaf partners as well. They took this to be one measure that *"people in the core of our community are facing the issue of violence in their lives"* (Merkin & Smith 1995:106). This service was also able to report that more cases were going to court as their public relations work reached out through workshops to community groups. A special focus on one group should not lead specialist services to become insular because they also play an important role in relation to mainstream agencies such as the police and criminal justice systems, which also need to initiate change to become more responsive to all people who have been abused and seek redress. The Seattle service provided a model of how this outreach and campaigning role could be combined with their function as a service provider.

> *"We do not work in isolation. We are a member of many coalitions and are active in local and state domestic violence and sexual assault committees. Each staff person at one time or another is committed to system change. Although we encourage referrals to our agency we provide ongoing training with every domestic violence and sexual assault agency in the county so that these agencies are always prepared to serve deaf and deaf-blind victims ... and because we all share common funding, we generally do lobbying as a group. The mutual support and respect we have for one another in the end helps victims."* (Merkin & Smith 1995:101)

Other specialist services struggle to bridge the gaps and funding peculiarities of different systems. A specialist refuge for women with intellectual disabilities evaluated by McCarthy (2000) found it difficult to operate on the same model as a women's refuge. Originally it had been intended to operate on the basis of self-referral and short-term placement but because the women with intellectual disabilities were being funded by social services, it was not possible to keep options open for them in their previous placements as this would entail double fees. Moreover the women using the refuge displayed many challenging behaviours which needed a more focused set of interventions than those usually provided in women's refuges.

Offenders who are themselves disabled may also need specialised interventions and safeguards and their needs have been addressed in the United Kingdom and in the Netherlands through training materials and service provision. A specialist assessment and counselling service exists in the United Kingdom called RESPOND (see also Thompson & Brown 1998) which works with intellectually disabled victims and perpetrators of sexual abuse. Offenders need to be given specific safeguards and legal advocacy to protect them against incriminating themselves during an investigation. If convicted, vulnerable offenders also need protection whether in prison or other facilities. Several member states have systems which "divert" vulnerable offenders from the criminal justice to the psychiatric system where they may be held in secure and/or closed placements (in the Flemish community in Belgium these are referred to as "social defence establishments"; in the United Kingdom as Special Hospitals or Secure Units). Terms of incarceration may be comparatively more lengthy in this parallel system and safeguards are needed to ensure that mentally disabled offenders are not disadvantaged in a system which is supposed to provide a more positive and rehabilitative ethos than prison. The European Committee for the Prevention of Torture and Inhuman or Degrading Treatment or Punishment (CPT 1998:12) comments on conditions in these facilities and also health care in prisons.

5.4.3. At government and community level

Tertiary prevention involves detailed planning of treatment options which are adapted to particular populations and which ensure that they receive at least as much support as other citizens who have been victimised. Where possible these services should be offered through mainstream agencies but where this is too complex then specialist provision must be set up. Creating a network of such provision requires long term planning and funding, including attention to disability equality awareness in the training of other professionals.

It is clear from this agenda that some tasks need to be addressed across national borders, including:

- Harmonising the conditions under which certain people will be excluded from the workforce;
- Sharing resources and expertise between all countries;
- Encouraging research and service development.

5.5. Summary

This chapter has explored the range of preventative measures which need to be in place to assure the safety of children and vulnerable adults. A model of prevention was presented which highlighted three dimensions:

- the stage of the intervention;
- the level at which such interventions are managed and implemented;
- the orientation either to empower service users and improve services proactively or to tackle abuse specifically through regulation and procedures designed to prevent potential abusers from entering the workforce.

Checklist

- Are initiatives in place to empower children and vulnerable adults through educational and advocacy programmes including education about rights and safeguards, sexual education and what constitutes abuse in the context of the services they use?
- Are service providers clear about their responsibility to recruit carefully and to train staff in how to respond positively to clients even when faced with difficult behaviours and complex needs?
- Is there a widespread commitment to user involvement and service user networks which are independent of service providers?

145

- Are treatment programmes and proper risk management in place to support, confront and contain, clients who are at risk of behaving violently to other children or vulnerable adults?

- Is detailed guidance available to staff about how to deal with challenging behaviour or emergency situations and about acceptable usage of control and restraint/ physical interventions?

- Is there legal advocacy available to people with disabilities and advocacy to assist them in accessing the criminal justice system?

- Is there an overarching policy document indicating how agencies are to work together when there are concerns about abuse of children with disabilities or vulnerable adults?

- Is there a coherent system of regulation and inspection in place to scrutinize the care offered to people with disabilities in institutions and residential homes?

- Is there a consistent system of professional regulation which lays out standards of good conduct and disciplinary/appeals procedures which allow individuals to be held accountable and removed from the workforce where there are reasonable concerns about their suitability to work with children or vulnerable people?

- Is it clear, and widely disseminated as to how concerns about abuse can be passed on and how referrals will be responded to?

- Are members of key agencies, eg the police, state prosecutors, social services, skilled in investigation and interviewing to obtain admissible evidence when harm has been done to a disabled child or adult?

- Is there a complaints system which can be easily accessed without jeopardizing the safety of a disabled child or adult?

- Are there special "places of safety" to which anyone at risk can be removed in an emergency?

146

- Is it clear to all professions in which circumstances they should override their usual rules about confidentiality in order to prevent abuse of disabled children or vulnerable adults?

- Are mainstream agencies (eg refuges, help lines and counselling services) which provide support to people who have been victimized trained and funded to provide services to disabled children and adults alongside other citizens?

- Is sensitivity to prior abuse built into assessment and service provision especially for people seeking help as a result of mental distress?

- Are services provided equitably to disabled children and adults from ethnic minority and refugee communities?

- Do governments sponsor regular audits of service provision and evaluation of treatment options for disabled children and adults who are recovering from abuses of their human rights?

The following template may be used to help policy makers to audit initiatives in their countries. Use a green pen for initiatives which are proactive and designed to empower service users or build good practice and a red pen for initiatives which have a more reactive focus and are specifically designed to avert the risk of abuse or bad practice. You may find it helpful to fill in a separate grid for children and adults and/or for each client group. You may then note gaps and discrepancies in protection for vulnerable children and adults.

Level of the initiative	Stage of intervention		
	preventing abuse from occurring at all	arrangements to ensure a prompt response	treatment and support in the aftermath of abuse
individual children and adults			
service providers (including mainstream agencies)			
Government and community			

6. RECOMMENDATIONS

6.1. Preface

This report has addressed issues of abuse against people with disabilities, making visible a broad range of harm and mistreatment, which occurs across a range of settings and circumstances. It advocates a model of protection, which does not cut across, but enhances the rights of disabled children and adults to take decisions and appropriate risks in their ordinary lives. As such the report builds on other agendas that are designed to support the empowerment of people with disabilities. This commitment sits alongside, and may be seen as part of, a wider commitment to integration and social inclusion as set out in the Council of Europe Recommandation on a Coherent policy for people with disabilities (Committee of Ministers of the Council of Europe 1992).

The report has offered a definition of abuse as a violation of human rights, which occurs against the backdrop of wider discrimination against, and exclusion of, disabled people across member states. It asserts the rights of people with disabilities (both children and adults) to be actively assisted in protecting themselves from harm, and where they are not able to do this unaided, it places a duty on member states to uphold their human rights and civil liberties. It documents how member states have tried, and often failed, to ensure equivalent protection for disabled people at law and in their use of service provision. It also embraces the concept of "equivalence" in access to health and personal care and identifies neglect and abandonment as significant threats to disabled citizens across member states. Addressing this agenda will involve ensuring access to mainstream provision and the creation of policies and service provision to specifically address the needs of people with disabilities.

The report has marshalled evidence, both anecdotal and scientific, to support the view that disabled children and adults are at considerable risk of abuse and mistreatment in all service settings (especially, but not exclusively, in large institutions), in their families or other accommodation and in their wider communities. This problem is not new but it is made newly visible because people with disabilities have spoken out about the way that they are treated and about the very widespread and pervasive discrimination that often underlies such mistreatment. Abuse often happens in services where staff are ill-equipped or poorly paid and where they pass on a feeling of resentment to those they are supposed to be assisting.

Where disabled people continue to be accommodated in large segregated institutions, their fundamental human rights may still be compromised including the fulfilment of basic needs such as nutrition, warmth, hygiene and privacy. Meanwhile, people with disabilities who live in more independent situations are insistent that they should be properly protected at least to the extent that other citizens are safeguarded

- within their local communities;
- in their dealings with professionals especially in the health care and criminal justice system; and
- in their contact with agencies which exist to support people who are victims of crime, domestic or personal violence.

Disabled people want the criminal justice system to be properly accessible to them and to hear their evidence without prejudice.

This report and the suggested initiatives outlined below will require action by government bodies and by NGO's and independent agencies representing disabled people, their families and carers. The balance of activity in each sector is likely to vary across member states depending on who currently organises service provision and on local arrangements for commissioning and monitoring services. What is essential is that there is collaboration between all agencies but that governments are clear that they remain centrally responsible for upholding the rights of disabled people as citizens of their countries even when they transfer some functions to non-statutory bodies.

Where independent NGOs take on the role of service provision they may compromise their position to campaign for safeguards in services. Service users who may need ongoing advocacy from genuinely independent bodies include those who are particularly vulnerable, for example those:

- with severe intellectual disabilities and/or challenging behaviours;
- who are subject to detention orders or are otherwise accommodated in secure settings and/or subject to compulsory treatment;
- who live in institutions;
- who live or work in settings/ neighbourhoods that may lead to their becoming the focus of hate campaigns or crimes.

Collaboration between service providers, networks of service users, academic and training institutions and government bodies are recommended as a way of providing such scrutiny and safeguards.

Although these recommendations focus primarily on people with disabilities, the framework we have produced may also be of use to agencies working with other vulnerable groups in society.

6.2. Recommendations to governments of member states

Governments are urged to draw up a programme of interrelated initiatives to assure the safety and protection of people with disabilities and provide access to redress where they are wronged. Checklists at the end of chapters on research, the legal framework and service provision provide additional instruments against which member states can evaluate their current practice and provision.

The working group recommends the following forms of action to prevent violence against disabled people.

6.2.1. Measures to facilitate further research

The working group recommends that international collaboration in research and service development should be strengthened and resourced appropriately and that this would be facilitated by

i.   Acknowledging risk of abuse in service settings and in the community and building this awareness into all research and service development programmes and protocols;

ii. Issuing standard definitions of disability and abuse;

iii. Mandating social welfare agencies to identify disabled children and adults within routine returns and statistics;

iv. Promoting research into incidence and prevalence of different types of abuse;

v.   Creating partnerships to conduct research across national boundaries;

vi. Stimulating research into, and evaluation of, service provision, especially in relation to difficult or controversial areas of practice such as behaviour modification, control, restraint and sexuality;

vii. Setting up research into, and evaluation of, professional education and training initiatives;

viii. Promoting research into multiple and complex needs, dual diagnoses and the most serious conditions including research into service provision to meet the needs generated by these conditions;

ix. Promoting research into treatments and interventions which are currently not acceptable to service users and/or which have damaging side-effects: for example seeking alternatives to ECT, aversive behavioural treatments and other irreversible interventions;

x.   Disseminating findings to all professional groups, including service managers and to unqualified staff, service users and their families, unpaid carers and volunteers, so that a consensus is built up about what are acceptable treatments and practices in relation to disabled children and adults.

6.2.2. Measures to promote the primary prevention of abuse

These recommendations build on an overarching commitment to anti-discriminatory practice both within health and social care services and across all public agencies and facilities. They are designed to **actively uphold human rights** and **assure opportunities for empowerment** by making service users safer and strengthening their position in the following ways.

a. *Information and assistance*

i. Providing educational campaigns for disabled children and adults outlining in an accessible form their rights, what acts and practices would constitute a breach of those rights and to whom they can complain if they are harmed or fear abuse in future;

ii. Providing educational programmes which teach disabled children and adults how to respect the rights of others;

iii. Providing appropriate support and assistance to families to help them care for their relatives in ways which respect their dignity, meet their needs and encourage empowerment;

iv. Stimulating changes in public attitudes and raising awareness to prevent discrimination and prejudice;

v. Making provision for a central well publicised help line with teletext and other accessible features to allow disabled people to report concerns to relevant authorities about service personnel in a form which guarantees their safety from reprisals and, if necessary, allows them to remain anonymous.

b. *Care and services*

i. Phasing out coercive and aversive techniques in behaviour modification, including time-out;

ii. Seeking and disseminating alternative, constructional approaches to such techniques wherever possible;

iii. Putting plans in place to reduce the size and/or increase the openness and accountability of institutionalized settings as well as assuring that the living standards in such institutions are comparable with those of the population in general;

iv. Ensuring that new forms of independent living include adequate safeguards, provisions for advocacy and social contact;

v. Making safer placements and groupings of clients using particular services so that service users who may abuse or be violent to others are not living alongside frail or vulnerable service users;

vi. Ensuring that disabled children and adults have access to a broad range of mainstream and independent service provision.

c. *Audit*

i. Encouraging groups of disabled people to comment independently on service provision;

ii. Introducing quality assurance systems and provision for independent audit and inspection into all settings in which disabled people receive services (including foster placements), which operate on the basis of explicit standards;

iii. Introducing stringent regulatory and monitoring activity where physical interventions and/or intrusive forms of surveillance are in operation;

iv. Introducing codes of conduct which are binding on both qualified and unqualified staff (whether paid or volunteer) to govern safe practice and reporting of abuse;

v. Implementing workable systems for screening of workers, for example through police checks, "certificates of good conduct" or the taking-up of references and where these are already in place for children extending them to settings which employ staff to work with vulnerable adults;

vi. Setting-up and supporting independent patient councils and user groups to provide advocacy to disabled people, including women's groups, gay and lesbian groups and groups for users from ethnic minorities including refugees;

vii. Monitoring of the health status of disabled people including provision of adequate nourishment and equivalent access to screening and preventative treatment;

viii. Setting-up and supporting of ethical committees to oversee and advise on controversial areas of practice.

d. Training

i. Promotion of training and of a well qualified and properly remunerated workforce;

ii. Expecting proper accountability in all services through supervision of staff and properly recorded shared decision-making and staff meetings;

iii. Supporting both qualifying and continuing training especially around difficult areas of practice;

iv. Providing training around disability and sexuality issues for all social workers, counselors, health care and mental health workers.

6.2.3. Measures to encourage prompt recognition, referral and investigation and prevent recurrence of abuse (secondary prevention)

These recommendations address the barriers that exist to recognition and reporting of concerns about abuse and also to the difficult balance which needs to be achieved between acting to protect vulnerable people and upholding the rights of those who might be implicated in harming them. These measures include:

a. Procedures for identifying and reporting potential abuse

i. Procedures for intervening in families when care is inadequate or restrictive;

155

ii   Providing programmes and information to help disabled people identify when they are being abused and know how to report their concerns;

iii. Setting-up of complaints systems and/or access to an ombudsperson which are monitored regularly: low usage of such procedures may not be an indicator that all is well in an establishment merely that dissent and concerns are stifled;

iv. Protection from dismissal or reprisals for "whistle-blowers" (employees who make public their concerns about poor standards or corruption in their workplace) both in statute and employment law and publicising of these safeguards in care settings.

b. *Sharing of sensitive information*

i.   Review of regulations about professional confidentiality with a special emphasis on the need to share information when vulnerable children or adults are at risk of abuse;

ii. Multi-agency guidance which indicates how member states intend that social welfare, health and criminal justice agencies will work together in cases involving harm to disabled children or adults;

iii. Member states should actively seek to reach agreement about the sharing of information necessary to protect vulnerable adults and children who move across local and national borders.

c. *Training*

i.   Providing training to all staff, volunteers and agencies on recognition of signs and symptoms of abuse;

ii. Putting in place structures for the training of all professionals involved, in how to conduct an impartial investigation of concerns and manage individual cases;

iii. Putting in place training for professionals in mainstream organisations with a special emphasis on workers in the criminal justice system, health care professions and staff working in therapeutic roles.

d. User involvement

i. Encouraging the inclusion of people with disabilities and their representatives (whether as professionals or lay people) on regulatory boards and inspection visits, tribunals and inquiry teams;

ii. Consulting disabled people and their organisations about child and adult protection and seek their suggestions for improvements to the system on a regular basis;

iii. Assuring the participation of disabled children and adults as victims and witnesses in hearings, tribunals and inquiries.

e. Safeguards

i. Having emergency provision so that immediate safety can be assured, wherever possible by removing the alleged perpetrator and not the victim;

ii. Providing support to all victims and witnesses who are vulnerable or have reason to feel intimidated.

6.2.4. Provision of treatment for people who have been abused (tertiary prevention)

The working group is concerned that both specialist and mainstream services are offered appropriately and sensitively to disabled children and adults who are victims of abuse including:

a. Accessing mainstream provision

i. Assuring that all mainstream agencies with a responsibility for people who have been victims of abuse are aware that, and take seriously the responsibility to provide help to people with disabilities who are victims of abuse (including domestic and sexual violence);

ii. Ensuring that budgets allow for an increase in accessible buildings, communication aids and access to and through new technology, as a routine part of any strategic review of mainstream services in order to guarantee that these

157

agencies operate without discriminating against disabled people;

iii. Evaluating on a regular basis access arrangements, usage and user satisfaction in relation to these services.

b. *Specialist provision*

i. Providing safe places and specifically some women-only services, for example women-only mental health services for disabled women who have endured previous abuse;

ii. Developing sufficient services for people with disabilities who have been abused including some specialised refuges and therapeutic provision;

iii. Providing specialist services and safeguards for offenders who are disabled or vulnerable.

c. *Developing skills*

i. Developing professional skills amongst workers in mainstream services and therapeutic professions with some training delivered by people with disabilities;

ii. Providing funding and scholarships so that disabled people can train as counsellors for victims of abuse;

iii. Providing training around disability and sexual abuse issues for all social workers, counsellors, health care and mental health workers so that they can contribute to the recovery process;

iv. Promoting specific post-qualifying training to equip some professionals working in the disability field to develop special expertise in the treatment of victims of abuse.

6.2.5. Measures to strengthen legal protection for people with disabilities

The working group's recommendations are built on, and seek to extend the principle of equality before the law for all people with disabilities. Where contentious decisions are to be made, the primary principle will be that disabled people will make their own decisions and, only if they are unable to do so will these be made by others acting in their best interest. If a decision is to be taken to protect their interests against their wishes or if there is an issue of public safety, decisions must be made within a clear legal framework with provision for appeal. People with diabilities and their representatives need to be able to access the court and judicial decision-making without barriers being placed in their way.

a. *Safeguards*

i. Affirmation that disabled people should always give informed consent to treatment unless it is shown on the basis of a formal assessment that they lack capacity to do so;

ii. Mechanisms for consultation and proxy decision-making so that people who lack capacity to make their own decisions are assisted in obtaining equivalent preventative and curative health care, civic status as for example in getting married or divorced, and financial security through assistance in managing their affairs;

iii. Upholding the right to judicial review or an independent hearing when any intrusive or irreversible interventions are suggested, for example sterilisation or involvement in medical research;

iv. Independent review of compulsory detention and treatment orders;

v. Regulation and scrutiny of any control, restraint, sedation or other intrusive treatments particularly as these affect people who are involuntarily detained or unable to give their own consent;

vi. Particular protection for disabled people who have been convicted of offences and who are held whether within the criminal justice or psychiatric system where they might otherwise endure longer sentences, fewer opportunities for review or parole and more deprivation/isolation.

b. *Access*

i. Changes in the law, law enforcement and courtroom practice to address the difficulty of bringing cases to court;

159

ii. Admission of expert witness testimony which provides independent and informed assessment of the credibility of witnesses or victims with disabilities in order to strengthen the position of disabled people in court;

iii. Arrangements to ensure that disabled victims and witnesses are given a fair hearing in court including through extension of schemes involving legal or non-legal representatives, "confidants" or intermediaries.

7. REFERENCES

7.1. Council of Europe Documents

Committee of Ministers of the Council of Europe (1979). Recommendation concerning the protection of children against ill-treatment, No. R (79) 17.

Committee of Ministers of the Council of Europe (1985). Recommendation on violence in the family, No. R (85) 4.

Committee of Ministers of the Council of Europe (1990). Recommendation on social measures concerning violence within the family, No. R (90) 2.

Committee of Ministers of the Council of Europe (1991). Recommendation on sexual exploitation, pornography and prostitution of, and trafficking in, children and young adults, No. R (91) 11.

Committee of Ministers of the Council of Europe (1992). Recommendation No. R (92) 6 on "A coherent policy for people with disabilities".

Committee of Ministers of the Council of Europe (1993). Recommendation on the medico-social aspects of child abuse, No. R (93) 2.

Committee of Ministers of the Council of Europe (1999). Recommendation on principles concerning the legal protection of incapable adults, No. R (99) 4.

Directorate General III – Social Cohesion (2000). Towards a Baltic Action Plan against sexual abuse and exploitation of children: a model for Europe. Plan for active prevention: policy framework identifying risks, components for action, models of good practice. Document CDCS PC (2000) 4. Strasbourg.

Dubet, F. & Vettenburg, N. (1999). Violence in schools: awareness-raising, prevention, penalties. Symposium, Brussels, 26-28 December 1998. Strasbourg: Council of Europe Publishing.

Dubet, F. & Vettenburg, N. (1999). Bullying in schools, ISBN 92-871-3752-8. Strasbourg: Council of Europe Publishing.

European Committee for the Prevention of Torture and Inhuman or Degrading Treatment or Punishment (CPT) (1998). 8th General Report on the CPT's activities covering the period 1 January to 31 December 1997. CPT/Inf (98) 12. Strasbourg.

European Convention on Human Rights. European Treaty Series, No. 5. Strasbourg: Council of Europe.

European Social Charter, European Treaty Series, No. 35. Strasbourg: Council of Europe.

Group of Specialists for Combating violence against women (EG-S-VL) (1997). Final report on the activities of the EG-S-VL including a Plan of Action for combating violence against women. EG-S-VL (97) 1. Strasbourg.

Oakley, R. (1996). *Tackling racist and xenophobic violence in Europe: review and practical guidance.* Strasbourg: Council of Europe Publishing.

Parliamentary Assembly of the Council of Europe (1998). Recommendation on abuse and neglect of children, R 1371 (1998).

Parliamentary Assembly of the Council of Europe (2000). Recommendation on violence against women in Europe, R 1450 (2000).

Study Group on Violence against Elderly People (1993). *Violence against elderly people.* Strasbourg: Council of Europe Press.

Working Party of the Steering Committee on Bioethics (2000). "White Paper" on the protection of the human rights and dignity of people suffering from mental disorder, especially those placed as involuntary patients in a psychiatric establishment. DIR/JUR (2000) 2. Strasbourg.

For further information on Council of Europe documents, please consult the following websites:

http://book.coe.int

www.coe.int

7.2. General References

ABCD Pack – Abuse and children who are disabled (1993). Training manual on protection for children with disabilities. ABCD Consortium.

AEP – Association Européenne de Psychiatrie (2000). Violences sur les handicapés. Présentation au Conseil de l'Europe, 30 mars 2000, Strasbourg.

Agthe Diserens, C. (1995). Des maux cachés aux mots pour le dire. Conférence inaugurale de la journée de réflexion du 21 avril 1995 sur la maltraitance et l'abus en milieu institutionnel accueillant des personnes handicapées.

Agthe Diserens, C. & Vatré, F. (2000a). "Du coeur au corps, formons-nous, puis... formons-les! " Prix Suisse 2001 de Pédagogie Curative. Programme de formation pour professionnels de l'éducation et de l'enseignement spécialisés ainsi que des soins.

Agthe Diserens, C. & Vatré, F. (2000b). *La sexualité et le(s) handicap(s)* – Dossier 69: Le handicap mental – enfants et adolescents; maltraitance et handicap. Lucerne: Edition SZH.

AIMS Project (1998). *The Alerter's Guide & Training Manual* and *The Investigator's Guide & Training Manual.* Brighton: Pavilion Publishing.

Alonso, M.A.V., Bermejo, B.G., Zurita, J.F., & Simón, J. A. E. (1994). *Maltrato infantil y minusvalía.* Madrid: Ministerio de Asuntos Sociales, INSERSO.

American Psychiatric Association (1994). *Diagnostic and Statistical Manual of Mental Disorders,* 4th ed. Washington DC.

ARC/NAPSAC (1993). It could never happen here: the prevention and treatment of sexual abuse of adults with learning disabilities in residential settings. Chesterfield ARC.

Australian Bureau of Statistics (1986). Victims of Crime Australia AGPO. Cited in Johnson, K., Andrew, R. & Topp, V. (1988), *Silent victims: a study of people with intellectual disabilities as victims of crime.* Victoria: Office of the Public Advocate.

Belie, E. de, Ivens, C., Lesseliers, J. & Hoven, G. van (2000). Sexual abuse of people with learning disabilities: prevention and assistance. MPI.

Bergh, P.M. van den, Hoekma, J. & Ploeg, D. van der (1997). Case file research: the nature and gravity of sexual abuse and the work method of an advisory team. *NAPSAC Bulletin,* 18, 16-21.

Bergh, P.M. van den, Douma, J. & Hoekema, J. (1999). *Zedenzaken en verstandelijk gehandicapten.* Leiden: DWSO Press.

Berlo, W. van (1995). *Seksueel misbruik bij mensen met een verstandelijke handicap: een onderzoek naar omvang, kenmerken en preventiemogelijkheden.* Delft: Eburon.

Brown, H. (1993). Sexuality and intellectual disability: the new realism. *Current Opinion in Psychiatry,* 6 (5), 623-8.

Brown, H. (1994). Lost in the system: acknowledging the sexual abuse of adults with learning disabilities. *Care in Place.* 1 (2), 145-57.

Brown, H., Egan-Sage E., Barry G. & McKay, C. (1996). *Towards better interviewing: a handbook for police officers and social workers on the sexual abuse of adults with learning disabilities.* "Need to know" Series. Nottingham: NAPSAC.

Brown, H. & Stein, J. (1997). Sexual abuse perpetrated by men with learning disabilities: a comparative study. *Journal of Intellectual Disabilities Research,* 41 (3), 215–24.

Brown, H. & Stein, J. (1998). Implementing Adult Protection Policies in Kent and East Sussex. *Journal of Social Policy,* 27 (3), 371–96.

Brown, H. & Stein, J. (2000). Monitoring adult protection referrals in ten English local authorities. *Journal of Adult Protection* 2 (3), 19-32.

Brown, H., Stein, J. & Turk, V. (1995). The sexual abuse of adults with learning disabilities: report of a second two-year incidence survey. *Mental Handicap Research,* 8 (1), 3-24.

Brown, H. & Thompson, D. (1997a). The Ethics of Research with Men who Have Learning Disabilities and Abusive Sexual Behaviour: a minefield in a vacuum. *Disability and Society,* 12 (5), 695–707.

Brown, H. & Thompson, D. (1997b) Service Responses to Men with Intellectual Disabilities who have Sexually Abusive or Unacceptable Behaviours: the Case Against Inaction. *Journal of Applied Research in Intellectual Disability,* 10 (2), 176–97.

Brown, H. & Turk, V. (1992). Defining sexual abuse as it affects adults with learning disabilities. *Mental Handicap,* 20 (2), 44-55.

Buckinghamshire County Council (1998), Independent Inquiry into LongCare Ltd, Aylesbury, England.

Cachemaille, Marguerite (2000). Autisme et violence: Position de l'Association Suisse romande de Parents d'Enfants autistes. *Pages Romandes – Revue d'information sur le handicap mental et la pédagogie specialisée,* 1, 10.

Cambridge, P. (1999). The first hit: a case study of the physical abuse of people with learning disabilities and challenging behaviour in a residential service. *Disability and Society* 14 (3), 285-308.

Cambridge, P. & Carnaby, S. (2000). *Make it personal: a training manual on intimate care.* Brighton: Pavilion Publishing.

CCMT – Commission cantonale vaudoise de prévention des mauvais traitements envers les enfants (1999). Concept de prise en charge et de prévention des mauvais traitements envers les enfants et les adolescents. Lausanne : Service de protection de la jeunesse.

Churchill, J., Brown, H., Craft, A., & Horrocks, C. (1997). There are no easy answers: the provision of continuing care and treatment to adults with learning disabilities who sexually abuse others. Chesterfield: ARC/NAPSAC.

Cohen, S. & Warren, R. (1990). The intersection of disability and child abuse in England and the United States. *Child Welfare* LXIX (3), 253-62.

Cooke, P. (1999). Summary of final report on disabled children and abuse. Ann Craft Trust, University of Nottingham.

Crosse, S.B., Kaye, E. & Ratnofsky, A.C. (1993). A report on the maltreatment of children with disabilities. Washington DC: National Center on Child abuse and Neglect.

Daniels, R.S., Baumhover, L. & Clark-Daniels, C. (1989). Physicians' mandatory reporting of elder abuse. *The Gerontologist,* 29 (3), 321-7.

Davies, C. & Beach, A. (2000). *Interpreting professional self-regulation: a history of the United Kingdom Central Council for Nursing, Midwifery and Health Visiting.* London: Routledge.

Davies, G. & Wilson, C. (1997). "Implementation of the memorandum: an overview ". In Westcott, H. & Jones, J. (1997), *Perspectives on the Memorandum: policy, practice and research in investigative interviewing.* Aldershot: Arena.

Defensor del Pueblo (1996). Estudio y recomendaciones del defensor del Pueblo sobre la atención residencial a personas discapacitadas y otros aspectos conexos. Madrid.

Delville, J. & Mercier, M. (1997). *Sexualité, vie affective et défi-cience mentale.* Paris: De Boeck Université.

Delville, J., Mercier, M. & Merlin, C. (2000). *Des femmes et des hommes : programme d'éducation affective, relationnelle et sexuelle destiné aux personnes déficientes mentales. Manuel d'animation, dossier d'images, vidéogramme.* Namur : Presses Universitaires de Namur.

Département de la prévoyance sociale et des assurances – Commission "Maltraitance et Handicap" (1996). Aspect – Respect – Conséquences du cadre légal concernant la maltrai-tance des personnes handicapées. Actes du colloque du 26.1.1996. Lausanne.

Département de la prévoyance sociale et des assurances – Commission "Maltraitance et Handicap" (1997). Soin de la violence : violence du soin. Actes du colloque du 16.4.1997. Lausanne.

Département de la prévoyance sociale et des assurances – Commission "Maltraitance et Handicap" (1998). Ethique et handicap : de l'illusion des discours à la confusion des pra-tiques. Actes du colloque du 22.4.1998. La Longeraie, Morges.

Department of Health (2000). No secrets: guidance on devel-oping and implementing multi-agency policies and proce-dures to protect vulnerable adults from abuse. London.

Department of Health (1999a). Report of the Expert commit-tee: review of the Mental Health Act 1983. London.

Department of Health (1999b). Quality Protects: Management Action Plans in relation to children with disabilities. London: SSI.

Diederich, N. (1998). Stériliser le handicap mental? Ramonville-Saint-Agne : Erés.

Doren, B., Bullis, M., & Benz, M. (1996). Predictors of victim-ization experiences of adolescents with disabilities in transi-tion. *Exceptional children,* 63 (1), 7-18.

167

Down, C. & Craft, A. (1997). *Sex in context.* Brighton: Pavilion Publishing.

Dyer, C. (2001). "Take your life in your own hands: that's my philosophy", *Guardian*, 6 March 2001.

European Commission (1999). European Day of Disabled People 1999 "Violence and Disabled People – root causes and prevention". Conference Report, 3 Dec 1999, Brussels.

European Disability Forum (EDF) (1999a). Report on violence and discrimination against disabled people. EDF 99/5. Brussels.

European Disability Forum (EDF) (1999b). How Article 13 Directives can combat disability discrimination. EDF 99/13. Brussels.

Evans, R. (2001). Inquiry into Cardiac Surgery Department, Royal Brompton Hospital, London. Cited in Kamal, A., "Doctors Deny Down's babies care", *Observer*, 1 April 2001.

Foubert, A. (1998). "Risk factors inherent in the structures of institutions and staff working in them". In *Autism Europe (1998), Code of Good Practice on Prevention of Violence against persons with autism.* Brussels.

Fovargue, S., Keywood, K. & Flynn, M. (1999). *Best practice? Health Care Decision-making by, with and for people with learning disabilities.* National Development Team and Joseph Rowntree Foundation.

Gabel, M. (1996). "Diversité, complémentarité et partenariat des professionnels". Dans Glatz, G. & Korpès, P. (1996), Etats généraux de la maltraitance: prise en charge multidisciplinaire et pratiques de réseaux, Congrès, 7.6.1996, Lausanne.

Garrett, T. (1998). Sexual contact between patients and psychologists. *The Psychologist,* 11 (5), 227-30.

Glaser, P. & Bentovim, A. (1979). Abuse and risk to handicapped and chronically ill children. *Child Abuse and Neglect,* 3, 565-75.

Goffman, E. (1961). *Asylums.* Harmondsworth: Penguin.

Gooding, C. (1998). Human Rights Violations and Disabled People: report prepared for the DPI Europe Human Rights Network project. London: DPI.

Hall, K.J. & Osborn, C.A. (1994). The conduct of socially sensitive research: sex offenders as participants. *Criminal Justice and Behaviour,* 21, 325-40.

Hardiker P., Exton, K., & Barker, M. (1995). The Prevention of Child Abuse: a framework for analysing services. London: NSPCC.

Harris, J. (1996). Physical restraint procedures for managing challenging behaviours presented by mentally retarded adults and children. *Research in Developmental disabilities,* 17 (2), 99-134.

Harris, J., Allen, D., Cornick, M., Jefferson, A. & Mills, R. (1996). Physical Interventions: a policy framework Kidderminster: BILD/National Autistic Society.

Hendey, N. & Pascall, G. (1998). Independent Living: gender, violence and the threat of violence. *Disability and Society,* 13 (3), 415-27.

Henley, J. (2000a). "Disabled girls secretly sterilised". *Guardian*, 12 September 2000, 17.

Henley, J. (2000b). "French kidnapper to get off, because he admits murder". *Guardian*, 16 December 2000, 19.

Hermansson, A., Hornquist, J. & Timpka, T. (1996). The wellbeing of war wounded asylum applicants and quota refugees following arrival in Sweden. *Journal of Refugee Studies,* 9 (2),166-81.

Hetherington, P. (2000). "Employers flout spirit of minimum wage law report". *Guardian*, 26 July 2000, 7.

Home Office, Department of Health, Department of Education and Science & Welsh Office (1989). Working together under the Children Act 1989: a guide to arrangements for interagency co-operation for the protection of children from abuse. London: HMSO.

Home Office & Department of Health (1992). Memorandum of Good Practice: video recorded interviews with child witnesses for criminal proceedings. London: HMSO.

Home Office (1998). Speaking up for Justice: report of an interdepartmental working group on the treatment of vulnerable or intimidated witnesses in the criminal justice system. London.

Home Office (1999). Action for Justice: implementing the Speaking up for Justice Report on vulnerable or intimidated witnesses in the Criminal Justice system in England and Wales. London.

Huizen, R.S. van, Visser, E.M., Vros, A.C. & Wisse, S.C. (1998). Pesten: een extra handicap: een exploratief onderzoek naar de beleving van pesten bij lichamelijk gehandicapte en/of chronish zieke kinderen in de leeftijd van 10 tot 15 jaar [Bullying: an extra handicap? An explorative study of the perseption of bullying of physically handicapped and/or chronically ill children between the ages of 10-15 years.] University of Utrecht: Wetenschapswinkel Sociale wetenschappen.

Jaudes, P. and Diamond, L. (1985). The handicapped child and child abuse. *Child Abuse and Neglect* 9, 341-7.

Kaplan, S., Pelcovitz, D., Salzinger, S., Weiner, A., Mandel, F., Lesser, M. & Labruna, V. (1998). Adolescent physical abuse: risk for adolescent psychiatric disorders. *American Journal of Psychiatry,* 155 (7), 954-9.

Kvam, M.H. (2000). Is sexual abuse of children with disabilities disclosed? A retrospective analysis of child disability and the likelihood of sexual abuse among those attending Norwegian Hospitals. *Child Abuse and Neglect,* 24 (8), 1073-84.

Law Commission (1995). Mental Incapacity. Law Commission Report No 231. London: HMSO.

Lee-Treweek, G. (1994). Bedroom abuse: the hidden work in a nursing home. *Generations Review,* 4 (1), 2-4.

Luckasson, R. (1992). People with mental retardation as victims of the criminal justice system. In Conley, R.,

Luckasson, R. & Bouthilet, G. (1992), *The criminal justice system and mental retardation: defendants and victims.* Baltimore: Paul Brookes.

Lyon, C. (1994). *Legal issues arising from the care, control and safety of children with learning disabilities who also present severe challenging behaviour.* London: Mental Health Foundation.

Marchant, R. & Page, M. (1992). *Bridging the gap: child protection work with children with multiple disabilities.* London: NSPCC.

Marchant, R. & Page, M. (1997). The Memorandum and disabled children. In Westcott, H. & Jones, J. (1997), *Perspectives on the Memorandum: policy, practice and research in investigative interviewing.* Aldershot: Arena.

Maroger, D. (1999). "Wounded Wombs" – a short film on the forced sterilisation of disabled women in France submitted to European Day of Disabled People Short Film Competition, Brussels 2 December 1999.

Maslow, A. H. (1943). A theory of human motivation. *Psychological Review,* 50 (4), 370-96.

McCarthy, M. (2000). An evaluative research study of a specialist women's refuge. *Journal of Adult Protection,* 2 (2), 29-40.

McCarthy, M. & Thompson, D. (1997). A prevalence study of sexual abuse of adults with intellectual disabilities referred for sex education. *Journal of Applied Research in Intellectual Disability,* 10 (2).

McCarthy, M. & Thompson, D. (1998). *Sex and the three rs: rights, responsibilities and risks.* Second Edition. Brighton: Pavilion Publishing.

McCreadie, C. (1996). Update on Research in Elder Abuse. London: Age Concern Institute of Gerontology, Kings College.

Mencap (1999). *Living in fear: the need to combat bullying of people with a learning disability.* London: Mencap.

171

Merkin, L. & Smith, M. (1995). A community based model providing services for deaf and deaf-blind victims of sexual assault and domestic violence. *Sexuality and disability,* 13 (2).

Ministère de l'emploi et de la solidarité (1998). Situations de maltraitance en institutions sociales et médico- sociales – Document de statistiques. Paris.

Ministère de l'emploi et de la solidarité (1999). Prévenir, repérer et traiter les violences à l'encontre des enfants et des jeunes dans les institutions sociales et médico-sociales: guide methodologique à l'attention des Médecins Inspecteurs de Santé Publique et des Inspecteurs des Affaires Sanitaires et Sociales. Paris.

Ministère de l'emploi et de la solidarité (2000). Prévenir, repérer et traiter les violences à l'encontre des enfants et des jeunes dans les institutions sociales et médico-sociales. Paris.

Ministerio de Trabajo y Asuntos Sociales (1997). Action plan for people with disabilities 1997-2002. Madrid: Instituto de Migraciones y Servicios Sociales.

Moody, H. (1988). From informed consent to negotiated consent. *The gerontologist,* 28 (suppl.), 64-70.

Moody, S. (1999). Protecting the vulnerable and including the marginal: volunteers and the law. *Journal of Adult Protection,* 1 (2), 6-16.

Murphy, G. (1997). "Treatment and risk management". In Churchill, J., Brown, H., Craft, A. & Horrocks, C. (1997), There are no easy answers. Chesterfields: ARC/NAPSAC.

Murphy, G. & Clare, I.C.H. (1995). "Adults' capacity to make decisions affecting the person: the psychologists' contribution". In Bull, R. & Carson, D. (1995), Handbook of Psychology in Legal Contexts. Chichester: Wiley.

Netto, G. (1998). "I forgot myself": the case for the provision of culturally sensitive respite services for minority ethnic carers of older people. *Journal of Public Health Medicine,* 20 (2), 221-6.

Ortega, G., González, J. & Cabanillas, M. (1997). Actitudes de los Españoles ante el Castigo Físico Infantil. Madrid: Ministerio de Trabajo y Asuntos Sociales.

Parens, E. & Asch, A. (2000). *Prenatal testing and disability rights.* Washington DC: Georgetown University Press.

Penfold, S. (1998). Sexual abuse by health professionals. Toronto: University of Toronto Press.

Pilgrim, D. (1995). "Explaining abuse and inadequate care". In Hunt, G. (1995), *Whistle-blowing in the Health Service: accountability, law and professional practice.* London: Edward Arnold.

Pillimer, K. & Finkelhor, D. (1988). The prevalence of elder abuse: a random sample survey. *The Gerontologist,* 28, 51-7.

Read, S. (1998). The palliative care needs of people with learning disabilities. *International Journal of Palliative Nursing,* 4 (5), 246-50.

Rioux, M. & Bach, M. (1994). *Disability is not measles.* Ontario: Roeher Institute.

Roberts, K. (2000). Lost in the system? Disabled refugees and asylum seekers in Britain. *Disability and Society,* 15 (6), 943-8.

Roeher Institute (1994). *Violence and people with disabilities: a review of the literature.* Ottawa: National Clearinghouse on Family Violence.

Rose, S., Peabody, C. & Stratigeas, B. (1991). Undetected abuse amongst intensive case management clients. *Hospital and Community Psychiatry,* 42 (5), 499-503.

Schoener, G. R., Milgrom, J.H., Gonsoriek, J.C., Luepker, E.T. & Conroe R.M. (1989). *Psychotherapists' sexual involvement with clients: intervention and prevention.* Minneapolis Walk in Counselling Center.

Sobsey, R. (1994). *Violence and Abuse in the Lives of people with disabilities.* Baltimore: Paul H. Brookes.

173

Sorheim, T.A. (1998). *Ordinary women – extraordinary challenges.* Oslo: University of Oslo, Department of Medical Anthropology.

Spencer, J.R. (1997). "The Memorandum: an international perspective". In Westcott, H. & Jones, J. (1997), *Perspectives on the Memorandum: policy, practice and research in investigative interviewing.* Aldershot: Arena.

Staffordshire County Council (1991). *The Pindown experience and the protection of children.* Staffordshire County Council.

Stanko, E. (2000). "Rethinking violence: rethinking social policy". In Lewis, G., Gerwitz, S., & Clarke, J. (2000), *Rethinking social policy.* London: Open University/Sage.

Stevenson, O. (1996). *Elder protection in the community: what can we learn from child protection.* London: ACIOG, Kings College.

Stewart, O. (1993). Double oppression: an appropriate starting point? In Swain, J., Finkelstein, V., French, S. & Oliver, M. (1993), *Disabling barriers – enabling environments.* London: Sage.

Swedish Social Services Department (1998). Social Services Act. Stockholm.

Terstegen, C., Hoekman, J. & Bergh, P. van den (1998). Behandeling en begeleiding na seksueel misbruik: een inventariserend onderzoek naar mogelijkheden voor behandeling en begeleiding voor verstandelijk gehandicapte slachtoffers en plegers van seksueel misbruik [Research report on Forms of treatment after sexual abuse for perpetrators or victims with intellectual disabilities]. Leiden: Universiteit Leiden, Afdeling Orthopedagogiek.

Thompson, D. (1997). A profile of sexual abusing behaviour by men with intellectual disabilities. *Journal of Applied Research in Intellectual Disability,* **10** (2).

Thompson, D. & Brown, H. (1998). *Response-ability: working with men with learning disabilities who have abusive or unacceptable sexual behaviours.* Brighton: Pavilion Publishing.

174

Tilley, C.M. (1998). Health Care for Women with Physical Disabilities: Literature Review and Theory. *Sexuality and Disability,* 16 (2), 87-102.

Turk, V. & Brown, H. (1993). The sexual abuse of adults with learning disabilities: results of a two-year incidence survey. *Mental Handicap Research,* 6 (3), 193-216.

UNAPEI – Union nationale des associations de parents et amis de personnes handicapées mentales (2000). Livre Blanc – Maltraitance des personnes handicapées mentales dans la famille, les institutions, la société ; Prévenir, repérer, agir. Paris.

Valentine, D. (1990). Double jeopardy: child maltreatment and mental retardation. *Child and Adolescent Social Work,* 7 (6).

Verdugo, M., Bermejo, B., & Fuertes, J. (1995). The maltreatment of intellectually handicapped children and adolescents. *Child Abuse & Neglect,* 19 (2), 205-15.

Vizard, E., Monk, E. & Misch, P. (1995). Child and Adolescent Sexual Abuse Perpetrators: a review of the research literature. *Journal of Child Psychology and Psychiatry,* 36, 731-56.

Vizard, E., Wynick, S., Hawkes, C., Woods, J. & Jenkins, J. (1996). Juvenile Sex Offenders: assessment issues. *British Journal of Psychiatry,* 168, 259-62.

Wade, A. & Westcott, H. (1997). "No easy answers: children's perspectives on investigative interviews". In Westcott, H. & Jones, J. (1997), *Perspectives on the Memorandum: policy, practice and research in investigative interviewing.* Aldershot: Arena.

Ward, L. (2001). Considered choices? The new genetics, pre-natal testing and people with learning disabilities. Kidderminster: BILD.

Wardhaugh, J. & Wilding, P. (1993). Towards an analysis of the corruption of care. *Critical Social Policy,* 37, 4-31.

Waterhouse Inquiry (2000). Report of the Tribunal of Inquiry into Child Abuse in North Wales. London: HMSO.

Welsh Office (2000). In safe hands: protection for vulnerable adults from abuse. Cardiff: SSI.

Westcott, H. (1991). The abuse of disabled children: a review of the literature. *Child care, health and development,* 12, 243-58.

Westcott, H. (1993). Abuse of children and adults with disabilities. London: National Society for Prevention of Cruelty to Children.

Westcott, H. & Jones, J. (1997). Perspectives on the Memorandum: policy, practice and research in investigative interviewing. Aldershot: Arena.

Westcott, H. & Jones, D. (1999). Annotation: the abuse of disabled children. *Child Psychology and Psychiatry,* 40 (4), 497-506.

Williams, C. (1993). Vulnerable victims? A current awareness of the victimisation of people with learning disabilities. *Disability, Handicap and Society,* 8 (2), 161-72.

Williams, C. (1995). *Invisible Victims: Crime and abuse against people with learning disabilities.* London: J. Kingsley.

Williams, C. & Evans, J. (2000). *Visible victims: the response to crime and abuse against people with learning disabilities.* Joseph Rowntree Foundation.

Wilson, C. & Brewer, N. (1992). The incidence of criminal victimisation of individuals with an intellectual disability. *Australian Psychologist,* 27 (2), 114-7.

Wolf, R. & Donglin, L. (1999). Factors affecting the rate of elder abuse reporting to a State Protective Services Program. *The Gerontologist,* 39 (2), 222-8.

Wolf, R. & Pillimer, K. (1994). What's new in elder abuse programming? Four bright ideas. *The Gerontologist,* 14 (1), 126-9.

Wolfensberger, W. (1987). *The new genocide of handicapped and afflicted people.* New York: Syracuse University.

Yuille, J. (1988). Credibility Assessment. Dordrecht: Netherlands Kluwer Academic Publishers.

Zijdel, L. (1999). Disabled people and violence. In European Commission (1999), European Day of Disabled People 1999 "Violence and Disabled People – root causes and prevention". Conference Report, 3 Dec 1999, Brussels.

APPENDIX

Members of the Working Group on Violence against, and Ill-treatment as well as Abuse of People with Disabilities

BELGIUM

M. Michel DE HARENNE
Attaché
Service "Prestations collectives"
Service Bruxellois francophone des personnes handicapées
Rue du Meiboom, 14
B-1000 BRUXELLES
Tel.: (32) 2 209 33 21 / 32 03
Fax: (32) 2 219 47 67

Mᵐᵉ Maryse HENDRIX
Responsable du Service "Agrément"
des Services résidentiels et d'accueil de jour
Service "Accueil et Hébergement
des Personnes handicapées"
A.W.I.P.H. (Agence wallonne pour l'Intégration des
Personnes handicapées)
Rue de la Rivelaine, 21
B-6061 CHARLEROI
Tel.: (32) 71 20 57 05
Fax: (32) 71 20 51 10
E-mail: mhendrix@awiph.be
Web Site: http://www.awiph.be

M. Paul KEMPENEERS
Directeur
Service "Staff"
Fonds Flamand pour l'Intégration sociale

des Personnes handicapées
Avenue de l'Astronomie, 30
B-1210 BRUXELLES
Tel.: (32) 2 225 84 66
Fax: (32) 2 225 84 05
E-mail: Paul.Kempeneers@vlafo.be

ESTONIA

Mrs Vilja KUZMIN
(Chair for 1st, 2nd and 3rd meetings)
Senior Specialist
Social Protection Department
Ministry of Social Affairs of Estonia
Gonsiori 29
EE-15027 TALLINN
Tel.: (372) 6269 757
Fax: (372) 6269 743
E-mail: vilja@sm.ee
Web Site: http://www.sm.ee

Mrs Helve LUIK
Chairwoman
Estonian Chamber of the Disabled People
Gonsiori 29
EE-15027 TALLINN
Tel.: (372) 6269 952
Fax: (372) 6269 951

FRANCE

Mme Michèle CREOFF (Chair of 4th and 5th meetings)
Inspectrice des Affaires Sanitaires et Sociales
Direction de l'Action Sociale
Ministère de l'Emploi et de la Solidarité
1, place de Fontenoy
F-75350 PARIS 07 SP
Tel.: (33) 1 44 56 86 34
Fax: (33) 1 44 56 88 38

ITALY

Dr Natalia NICO FAZIO
Fonctionnaire
Servizio "Disabili"
Dipartimento per gli Affari Sociali
Presidenza del Consiglio dei Ministri
Via Veneto, 56
I-00187 ROMA
Tel.: (39) 06 48 16 13 35
Fax: (39) 06 48 16 13 39
E-mail: anziani@affarisociali.it

LUXEMBOURG

Mme Mir OESCH
Employée
Ministère de la Famille, de la Solidarité sociale et de la
Jeunese
Avenue Emile Reuter,
L-2919 Luxembourg
Tel.: (35) 2 478 65 99
E-mail: mirjam.oesch@fin.etat.lu

Mme Patricia WEICKER
Juriste
Département aux handicapés et accidentés de la vie
Ministère de la Famille, de la Solidarité Sociale
et de la Jeunesse
12-14, avenue Emile Reuter
L-2919 LUXEMBOURG
Tel.: (352) 478 6567
Fax: (352) 478 6570

THE NETHERLANDS

Mrs Marije SCHADEE
Policy Official
Directorate Policy for the Disabled
Ministry of Health, Welfare and Sport
P.O. Box 20350

NL-2500 EJ THE HAGUE
Fax: (31) 70 340 5371 / 7164
E-mail: me.schadee@minvws.nl

NORWAY

Ms Anne-Margrethe BRANDT
Head of Division
The State Council on Disability
P.O. Box 8192 DEP
N-0034 OSLO
Tel.: (47) 22 24 85 58
Fax: (47) 22 24 95 79
E-mail: anne-margrethe.brandt@srff.dep.no

Mr Alf HAGELIN
Legal Adviser
Department of Social and Health Care Policy
Ministry of Health and Social Affairs
Grubbegata 10
P.O. Box 8011 DEP
N-0030 OSLO
Tel.: (47) 22 24 85 67
Fax: (47) 22 24 27 66
E-mail: alf.hagelin@shd.dep.no

PORTUGAL

Mme Maria do Pilar MOURÃO-FERREIRA
Chef de Division
Cabinet des Relations Internationales et Affaires
Européennes
Secrétariat National pour la Réadaptation et l'Intégration des
Personnes Handicapées
Av. Conde Valbom, 63
P-1069-178 LISBOA
Tel.: (351) 1 792 95 79
Fax: (351) 1 797 26 42
E-mail: pilar.ferreira@snripd.mts.gov.pt

Mme Teresa BOTELHO
Psychologue
Centre d'Investigation et de Formation
Secrétariat National pour la Réadaptation et l'Intégration des
Personnes Handicapées
Av. Conde Valbom, 63
P-1069-178 LISBOA
Tel. (351) 1 940 64 18
Fax (351) 1 941 13 24

M. Adalberto FERNANDES
Assesseur
Cabinet du Secrétaire National
Secrétariat National pour la Réadaptation et l'Intégration des
Personnes Handicapées
Av. Conde Valbom, 63
P-1069-178 LISBOA
Tel. (351) 1 792 95 73
Fax (351) 1 796 51 82

SLOVENIA

Mr Damijan JAGODIC
Adviser
Government Office of the Republic of Slovenia for the
Disabled
Železna Cesta 14
7 SLO-1000 LJUBLJANA
Tel. (386) 61 17 35 538
Fax (386) 61 17 35 540
E-mail damjan.jagodic@gov.si

Mrs Biserka DAVIDOVIČ PRIMOŽIČ
Government Adviser
Government Office of the Republic of Slovenia
for the Disabled
Železna Cesta 14
SLO-1000 LJUBLJANA
Tel. (386) 61 17 35 522

183

Fax: (386) 61 17 35 525
E-mail: davidovic.biserka@gov.si

SPAIN

M. Gaspar CASADO GÓMEZ
Subdirección General del Plan de Acción y Programas para
Personas con Discapacidad
IMSERSO
Avda. de la Ilustración, c/v a Ginzo de Limia, 58
E-28029 MADRID
Tel.: (34) 91 347 8818
Fax: (34) 91 347 8855
E-mail: gcasadog@MTAS.es
Web Site: http://www.seg-social.es/imserso

Mrs Rosa Maria BRAVO RODRIGUEZ
Subdirección General del Plan de Acción y de
Programas para Personas con Discapacidad
IMSERSO
c/Ginzo de Limia, 58
E-28029 MADRID
Tel.: (34) 91 347 88 13
Fax: (34) 91 347 88 55

SWITZERLAND

M. Hannes SCHNIDER
Secrétaire Général
Entraide Suisse Handicap
Association AGILE, Behinderten-Selbsthilfe Schweiz
Effingerstr. 55
CH-3008 BERN
Tel.: (41) 31 390 39 39
Fax: (41) 31 390 39 35
E-mail: info@agile.ch
Web Site: http://www.agile.ch

Madame Catherine AGTHE DISERENS
Sexo-Pedagogue Spécialisée
14, ch. du Couchant

CH-1260 Nyon
Tel.: (41) 22 361 15 29
Fax: (41) 22 361 15 29
E-mail: catherine.agthe@bluewin.ch

Madame Susanne SCHRIBER
Zollikerstr. 238
CH-8008 Zürich
Tel.: (41) 1 383 8430

UNITED KINGDOM

Ms Annette YOUNG
Health and Social Care Consultant – Department of Health
99, Pembroke Road
Clifton
GB-BRISTOL BS8 3EE
Tel.: (44) 117 973 24 24 (Home)
Fax: (44) 117 974 16 74 (Home)
E-mail: ayoung@onetel.net.uk

COMMISSION OF THE EUROPEAN COMMUNITIES

Mme C LE CLERCQ
EMPL /E/4
J27 – 02/015
Commission Européenne
27 Rue Joseph II,
B-1040 BRUXELLES
Tel.: (32) 2 295 00 26
Fax: (32) 2 295 10 12
E-mail: Cecile.Leclercq@cec.eu.int

Mme Elena NIELSEN GARCIA
Administrateur
J27 – 00/122
Unité "Intégration des Personnes handicapées"
Direction Générale V/E/4
Commission Européenne
Rue de la Loi, 200
B-1049 BRUXELLES

Tel.: (32) 2 295 24 23
Fax: (32) 2 295 10 12
E-mail: elena.nielsen@bxl.dg5.cec.be

CONSULTANT

Prof Hilary Brown, PhD (Social Work)
Salomons
Canterbury Christ Church University College
Broomhill Road
Southborough
Nr Tunbridge Wells
GB-Kent TN3 0TG
Tel.: (44) 1892 507675
Fax: (44) 1892 507660
Website: www.salomons.org.uk

Sales agents for publications of the Council of Europe
Agents de vente des publications du Conseil de l'Europe

Council of Europe Publishing/Editions du Conseil de l'Europe
F-67075 Strasbourg Cedex
Tel.: (33) 03 88 41 25 81 – Fax: (33) 03 88 41 39 10 – E-mail: publishing@coe.int – Website: http://book.coe.int

CANCELLED